W9-BYZ-209

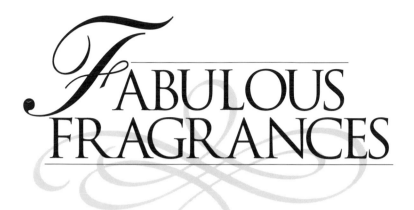

FABULOUS FRAGRANCES

HOW TO SELECT
YOUR PERFUME WARDROBE

THE WOMEN'S GUIDE TO PRESTIGE PERFUMES

JAN MORAN

CRESCENT HOUSE PUBLISHING
BEVERLY HILLS

Crescent House Publishing
P.O. Box 16724
Beverly Hills, CA 90209
(310) 364-0551

Design by Howard Yang and Sherri Yu/Wonder Studio

Library of Congress Cataloging-in-Publication Data
Moran, Jan.
   Fabulous fragrances: how to select your perfume
wardrobe, the women's guide to prestige perfumes / by
Jan Moran

CIP 93-90954

ISBN 0-9639065-5-0 (hardcover)

Disclaimer: In *Fabulous Fragrances* we (Crescent House
Publishing and Jan Moran) have relied on information
provided by third parties and have performed reasonable
verification of facts. While we believe that these sources
are reliable, we assume no responsibility or liability for
the accuracy of information contained in this book.
No representations or warranties, expressed or implied,
as to the accuracy or completeness of this book or its
contents are made. The information in this book is
intended for entertainment purposes only.

Every effort has been made to locate the copyright holders
of materials used in this book. Should there be any errors
or omissions, we apologize and shall be pleased to make
acknowledgements in future editions.

Note: Some components in perfumes may cause allergic
reactions, so reasonable care should be taken in use.
If symptoms arise, consult a physician.

FOREWORD

I am honored to have been invited to write a foreword to *Fabulous Fragrances* because it teaches and guides women through the maze of delectable fragrances on the market, empowering them to make the proper use of a potent, invisible form of communication. Jan Moran asked me to share my personal experiences in the world of fragrance, how I develop perfumes, and what makes them successful.

I believe that fragrance is ageless, as appealing to the young as to the mature. My own interest was sparked early, when as a young girl studying at the American School of Ballet in New York I used to buy fifteen-cent vials of perfume at Woolworth's. Little did I know that these golden liquids would shape my future.

A few years later, while married to Fred Hayman and in partnership with him as owners of the Giorgio Beverly Hills store, I researched trends in the world of fashion and fragrance and learned firsthand what women wanted. It was the 1970s, and change was in the air. At the store, we created total fashion concepts, from hats to gloves. It was only natural that a

fragrance should follow, for perfume is a fashion accessory, the last thing that goes on before your earrings.

Some of our Giorgio customers had vivid signature fragrances. For example, when the scent of Jungle Gardenia floated through the room, instinctively I would turn to look for Elizabeth Taylor or Natalie Wood.

When I created the Giorgio fragrance, I drew upon my experiences and the changing times. Fragrance, like art, is a reflection of the times. The women's movement was gaining momentum and women wanted equality, but they still wanted to be feminine and glamorous. I knew the fragrance would have to be both sensual and aggressive.

What did I look for then in a fragrance, and what do I still look for? Foremost, originality. Originality is the key. I look for a fragrance that doesn't smell like anything else. Next, the formula must be capable of becoming a classic, because classics set trends for others to follow. I can imagine, almost visualize a fragrance in my head—I can actually smell the notes—just as a

In loving memory of my brother,
Frank Hollenbeck,
and the music in his soul
November 24, 1953
to
December 31, 1993

For my mother, Jeanne,
whose love of perfume inspired me.
For the men in my life—
my son, Eric, and my husband, Jim.
For my cousin, Monique.

And for all who enjoy fabulous fragrances.

composer hears music. Finally, I look for elements that arrest your attention. Instinctive reactions. When that happens, I know it's right.

But even though I had spent more than two years searching and sampling, the magic still eluded me. Once when I was at lunch with Karl Lagerfeld I asked him how long it took him to create the Chloé fragrance. He said, "Darling, if it takes more than two years, forget it." Well, I didn't. And one day, the formula clicked and the Giorgio fragrance was born. The timing was perfect.

Now, ten years later, women can afford to relax with their work. We still work just as hard, but thanks to the women's movement and work place advances we don't have to fight as much. We have achieved. We feel comfortable wearing pink and running a company. Today, the symbol of my company is the leopard, which I believe is a fitting symbol for women today. We can be strong and assured, sleek and elegant. Our attitudes are changing, so in response I created my newest fragrance, Delicious, which you'll read more about in this book.

I love every minute of my work, all of it from A to Z, every nuance, every challenge. I work with chemists, perfumers and physicians in developing my fragrances as well as my skin care and makeup line. I prefer natural ingredients as much as possible, and I still visit fragrance counters anonymously to listen to what women are talking about, learning their likes and dislikes.

After I create one fragrance, I'm on to the next, like an artist who lives to paint. As you read, I think you'll enjoy experimenting with all the wonderful scents as much as I do. When you or those around you react instantly and say, "That smells fabulous!" you'll know you've got a hit.

Gale Hayman
Chief Executive Officer
Gale Hayman Beverly Hills

ACKNOWLEDGMENTS

It is impossible to succeed in a vacuum. I am indebted to a great many kind people who have graciously given of their time, information, assistance, and enthusiasm. May your kindness be returned in abundance.

My loving appreciation to my husband, Jim Halper, who was the first to say, "Write it!" when I lamented, "There ought to be a guide book for perfumes...." To Monique Schaeffer, who supports *almost* every idea, and who came on board with Crescent House Publishing to market and promote *Fabulous Fragrances*. To Suzie Yazzie, who somehow keeps me organized. To Aly Spencer and Peter Aynsley, for diverting my attention when it needed diverting.

My sincere thanks to Gale Hayman and Georgette Mosbacher, for their enthusiasm, support and role modeling. To Annette Green and the Fragrance Foundation staff, for their incomparable assistance.

For their gracious words of praise, my heartfelt appreciation to Elizabeth Taylor, Oleg Cassini, Bijan, Dr. Linda Hill and William Owen.

To Bunni Nance and Mary Ellen Van Der Wal at Neiman Marcus, for their invaluable information and friendship. To my heroine Frankie, who waited patiently in my then-unfinished novel while I perfected her perfume and wrote *Fabulous Fragrances*.

My appreciation to the many fragrance houses that contributed information and photography, including Benetton, Bijan, Boucheron, Bulgari, Caesars, Cassini, Chanel, Liz Claiborne, Classic Fragrances, Compar, Cosmair (Lancôme, Ralph Lauren, L'Oréal, and European Designers), Dionne Warwick, Erox, Escada, EuroCos, French Fragrances, Guerlain, Halston Borghese, Gale Hayman, Fred Hayman, Hermès, Lancaster, Jessica McClintock, Marilyn Miglin, Madeleine Mono, Niro, William Owen, Parfums International, Jean Patou, Prescriptives, Revlon, Riviera Concepts, Rochas, Paul Sebastian, Tiffany, Ungaro, Vepro, and others, without whom there would be no book.

To my editor Eileen Heyes, for her eagle eye and expertise. To the many wonderful people who divulged their favorite fragrances and those of their friends. To Patti Slesinger, David Benson and Sabra Chili for printing; to Howard Yang and Sherri Yu for design. To Ali Ferber for her technical assistance, and Douglas Olson for his photography.

Thanks and God bless y'all.

JM
Beverly Hills, 1994

CONTENTS

LIST OF
FRAGRANCE PROFILES

INTRODUCTION

FRAGRANT MEMORIES

For me, perfume always represented the luxurious life, a life to be lived to the fullest, not hoarded away for special occasions and future days. Life was a voyage and perfume was the passage. It was the olfactory key to a glamorous life far beyond the confines of my small Texas town. It was to my senses what books were to my soul: an avenue of escape to a grown-up F. Scott Fitzgerald world, a world where days were pretty and kind and sweet, and nights were sultry and languid and full of mysterious men. A world where each dawning day held the promise of glittering adventure.

I remember as a little girl, barely five years old, playing at my mother's old-fashioned vanity, the one with the large beveled mirror and two columns of drawers, where I would perch on the velvet-covered stool and sample her brilliant red lipsticks, finely-sifted face powders and youth-enhancing cremes. Then I would gaze at myself in the mirror, imagining the elegant, sophisticated woman I would surely grow to be.

But the *pièce de résistance*, the ultimate glory, was in her carved crystal decanters of perfume. I reveled in their exotic names: Shalimar, Bal à Versailles, Mitsouko, Arpège.

Whispering these names, I was whisked away to the streets of Paris, the palaces of India and the gardens of Japan, all filled with worldly people, mystery, romance and opulence. Then there were the names I could understand, like Youth Dew, Joy and Royal Secret. I remember the day when I learned to pronounce L'Air du Temps and Quelques Fleurs, and understood their meaning. I had unlocked a door; my voyage had begun.

It was before that mirror that I first experienced those fragrant creations. Of course, I had smelled them long before, on my mother and grandmother. My mother, who often smelled of Shalimar; my mother, who was different from every other mother, who to me was prettier and more refined and who never stepped out of the house without lipstick, never wore hair curlers in public. And my grandmother, who favored White Shoulders and never went out, not even to the grocery store or for a neighborhood walk, without her "face" on, her hair perfectly coiffed, makeup flawless. Even when she died at 86, she looked fabulous, much to her eternal relief, I'm sure.

The makeup was important, but the perfume was absolutely mandatory, even at home. Perfume was applied in the morning, touched up during the day, and added to the evening bath water. In a home that knew few luxuries, fragrance was deemed an essential, like milk and bread.

Perhaps it was because my mother was a ballet dancer, and she understood the necessity of art and romance in life. Or maybe it was because it brought back memories of my father, who died when I was seven, a man who had showered my mother with love and adoration, along with French perfume and couture clothes, and fancy boxed chocolates every month when it was "that time." The type of man it took me more than thirty years to find.

Whatever the reason behind my mother's and grandmother's love of fragrance, I understood it instinctively. I remember my mother would let me dab the precious oils on my wrists and neck, and spritz the eau de toilette lavishly on my hair and shoulders. Even on my Barbie dolls, who, after my father died, remained the only truly spoiled members of the household, with their extensive wardrobes handmade from remnant silks and satins. As a little girl I learned to distinguish the scents: the florals and spices, the greens and woods. I just didn't realize it until I was much older, when I would search for words to describe a scent. Instinctively I knew when and where to wear a fragrance: the spicy, rich, opulent scents for romantic dates; the fresh citrus and white flower eau de toilettes for daytime, for school, and for ballet class.

I assumed that everyone understood and enjoyed fragrance as I did. I always carried an assortment of petite perfume bottles—a practice that delighted my girlfriends, who quickly depleted my supply. Never would I travel

without selecting just the right scent, a fragrance light and not too overpowering for a confined airplane or train. No sooner would I venture out into the world without my tiny vials than would Napoléon have forged into battle without his saber. Or without his vats of eau de Cologne, a practice that inspired Guerlain scents and their famous "bee bottle" flacons, created in honor of the Emperor. Later, as a struggling student, I wouldn't dream of going to class without a suitable scent, even if I had just rolled out of bed with ten minutes to class time. The bare essentials were contact lenses, coffee and perfume. Now, I wouldn't even think of going to the gym without my miniature flacons to douse myself with after a workout. In the morning, the fragrance goes on right after I brush my teeth, even if I don't plan to leave the house or the garden that day.

Gardening, in fact, was another of my mother's and grandmother's passions. Perhaps it was the fragrance of the flowers and leaves. I remember the constant propagations, the herbs and gardenias and honeysuckle. The scented geraniums and heady roses. The fresh buds that made the peach and plum trees along our back fence look like popcorn trees in the spring. Texas, with its freezing winters and hot, humid summers, was not an easy place to grow plants. I remember shuffling plants indoors on frostbitten nights, and out again on sunny days; into the shade on a searing afternoon, out again on a summer night to catch the morning dew and soft sun.

Our home came to smell like a fragrant greenhouse. Gleaming vases of cut roses and gardenias scented every room in the spring and summer. And on Easter, I remember my mother pinning gardenias to my straw hat before church. To this day, I love gardenias; I have two pruned gardenia trees at my front door, just so I can catch a whiff as I enter or depart.

I garden by smell—jasmine, lantana, herbs, citrus trees. Imagine my disappointment to find a lovely camellia bush in my yard, laden with blooms but lacking in fragrance. Only to be appreciated from afar. Inside my home, my floral arrangements are chosen as much for fragrance as for color—eucalyptus, pine, roses, tuberose. Carnations and cedar, cinnamon and rinds of oranges, lemons and lime. I even dust my bed linens with powder and toss empty perfume flacons along with sachets in my lingerie drawers.

Fragrance weaves through my life like the silken tasseled cords that entwine my handblown perfume bottles. I still remember the smell of the cedar trees my father cut at Christmas, even though later I was found to be severely allergic to them. Just as I recall the smell of the cedar chest my grandmother kept in her back bedroom—it was much more agreeable to my sinuses than the fresh-cut Christmas tree.

Name a fragrance and memories flood back. Like Opium, the perfume an old boyfriend brought to me from French Martinique. Or Joy, the one another boyfriend gave me while we were in Hong Kong. Or Halston Z-14, the men's cologne a Hungarian soccer player boyfriend always wore—his closets and car reeked of it, and I loved it. For years I surreptitiously followed men who wore it out of elevators, basking in my memories. Then there was the Brut my brother Frank wore and the Old Spice my grandfather wore; the Aramis my

brother Mike wears. The Safari and Coco a girlfriend gave me before she moved from Beverly Hills, fragrances my husband likes so much on me. The Obsession another girlfriend gave me when I went to Harvard. The perfume I shan't name that I gave away, even though I loved it, when my husband said he hated it on me—I loved him so much more. The Lagerfeld he wears so well. The Shalimar that my mother wore, that I now wear when I feel nostalgic and romantic. Or the first Chanel No. 5 I was given as a teenager, the day when I felt really grown up. And more...the Bijan, the Delicious, the Fleurs de Rocaille...and the essences I blend today, always in search of a magical composition. Each fragrance is fraught with memories.

I remember when I hung up my toe shoes, packed my pastels, and shuffled away my stories, intent upon earning my living not as an artist but as an investment banker, which seemed a good way to support my son after my divorce. I put education first, studying business and finance. But I had to support myself in the interim, before I could dazzle Wall Street. Perfume came to my rescue.

I landed a variety of part-time jobs, as many as I could handle, working for fragrance companies. To Yves Saint Laurent, Oscar de la Renta, Anaïs Anaïs, Valentino, Perry Ellis, Lancôme, Alexandra de Markoff, Germaine Monteil and Guerlain I owe my University of Texas education, my B.B.A. in finance. I remember the photo I took on Santa's lap one Christmas, when I was dead tired from my last final. Immediately after the exam, I had donned a yellow satin jacket emblazoned with the word "Giorgio" and had gone to work in a department store, introducing the scent to scores of interesting people. There I met Santa Claus, and a photo with my yellow Giorgio jacket seemed appropriate. In Boston, my Harvard M.B.A. was partially financed by my work with Ralph Lauren, Claude Montana, Red, Paloma Picasso and a host of other fragrances. Case studies by night, perfume sales by day.

Upon graduation, I thought I'd leave the fragrance world far behind. But I soon found Wall Street and corporate America too repressive for my artistic soul. Something just didn't smell right. Before long, I had once again picked up my writing, my gardening and my perfumes, finally lured back to my senses.

A scientist once told me that our olfactory sense is our most retentive sense, a trigger for memory and emotion. Ancient cultures knew this and prized their fragrance and incense. Mystical, magical, mercurial. Today, perfume is produced from a combination of science, sense and business. So my return to the world of fragrance was perhaps inevitable, embedded as it was in my memory. But now, along with my innate appreciation and love of perfumery, I also have the tools to understand, create and manage fragrant endeavors.

Somewhere I read that within each of us is a divine plan waiting to unfold. Looking at my life, I can see a pattern. I understand how wonderful it is to be creative and productive, to use your senses and love what you do, each day of your life.

I love perfume, and I also adore the accoutrements of perfume. A person has to enjoy the trappings of her passions, as my hunter-fisherman husband favors camouflage and duck decoys. I love the opulent packaging,

the satin ribbons and golden seals, the fluffy powder puffs, and the glimmering array of colored crystal flacons reflected on my mirrored dressing shelves. I love the feel of a rich body creme, especially if it makes my skin sparkle in the sunlight. I love the glamorous scented bubbles in my morning bath water. I love the immediate confidence and poise garnered with each application, and the luxury of smelling the scent on the back of my hand in order to spark my imagination when I'm bored. I enjoy the total package and the ability to create, appreciate and share all the elements. It is my most enjoyable work, my voyage, my adventure.

I love the memories and I love the dreams, and most of all, I love the fragrances—part of the nuance and essence of life.

It is my hope that you will share a little part of my passion, like a sip of fine vintage wine. I welcome your comments and have provided a card for your response. If it is gone, you'll find the information on the last page. If you have information to share, I'd be delighted to include it in the next edition so that we might all benefit.

And in the spirit of sharing, a portion of *Fabulous Fragrances* profits will be donated to nonprofit organizations for breast cancer, AIDS and medical research through the Louis M. and Birdie Halper Foundation, a nonprofit entity organized and endowed by my husband's loving parents. Selected charities include the Dana-Farber Cancer Institute, the Revlon/UCLA Women's Cancer Research Program and the Elizabeth Taylor AIDS Foundation.

Jan Moran

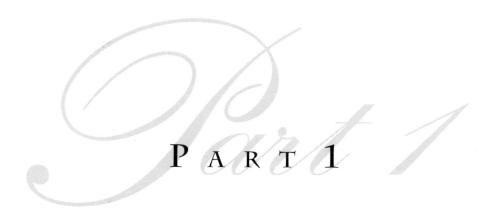

PART 1

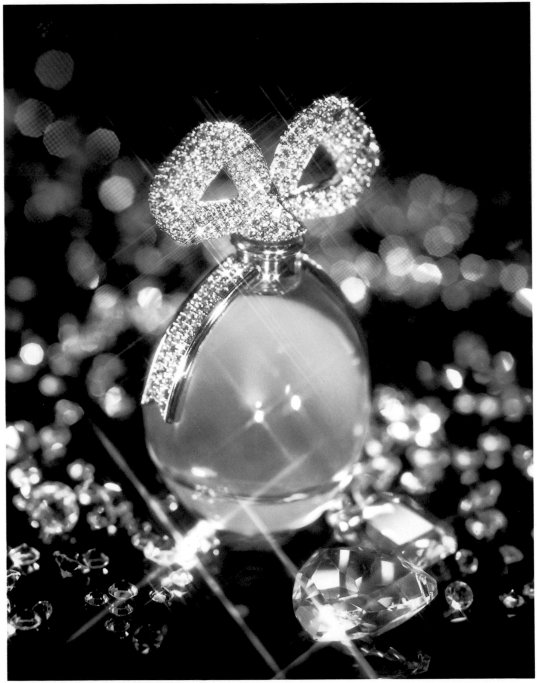

Elizabeth Taylor's White Diamonds

PERFUME

—the word conjures up images of romance, sensuality, power and style. Perfume cloaks a woman with mystery and confidence; it is the transparent veil that turns heads in her wake. Its allure is legendary; women from Cleopatra to Empress Josephine to Coco Chanel have treasured its magic.

The world of perfume is a world of art, a world of science. A compelling world based on our powerful sense of smell. Happily, it is also a world any woman can enter to find the fragrance to say, "This is who I am, my enjoyment, part of my image today."

Eighteenth-century philosopher Jean-Jacques Rousseau described this world well, saying, "Smell is the sense of the imagination."

To understand just how powerful and articulate your olfactory sense is, close your eyes for a moment and inhale deeply, slowly. Imagine the smell of a fireplace and the vision an evening spent in front of a fireplace will emerge; think of how fireworks smell and the picture a Fourth of July party may leap into your mind. Remember the smell of chalk, of baby powder, of a locker room, of a farm, of the ocean or of Christmas. Evocative memories, full of imagery. Some may be romantic, others painful. Jean Harlow's husband is said to have drenched himself with her favorite fragrance, Mitsouko, and then, in a fit of despair over their irreparable relationship, shot himself. On a happier note, Aimé Guerlain created the fragrance Jicky in honor of his first true love. But there is much more to finding the right fragrance than just taking a quick whiff at the perfume counter.

Perhaps the perfume you admire on a friend is horrid on you. Or your own favorites seem different in winter than in summer, different still when you're happy or angry, ill or well. Those differences aren't imaginary—weather, body chemistry and even mood can affect fragrance.

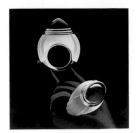

Boucheron

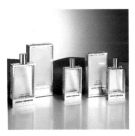

Calandre

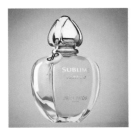

Sublime

How Do I Find the Right Perfume?

It may help to compare the selection of wine to the selection of fragrance. Indeed, there are many similarities—there are even vintages in perfume oils as there are in wines—so let's paint a picture.

First, imagine a chilly winter's evening, with a fire roaring in the fireplace and steaks broiling in the kitchen. In choosing a wine to go with dinner, you will consider the heaviness of the meal, steaks and baked potatoes, along with the chill in the air and your own preference. To balance the meal you may reach for a full-bodied red wine, say a Bordeaux or Burgundy, and serve it close to room temperature to warm your guests. After the meal, you might serve gently warmed cognac. But what if you don't like red wine, or you're allergic to it? Naturally, you'll choose another beverage, but you'll still consider the appropriateness. You probably wouldn't serve ice tea.

If you were selecting a fragrance for the same evening, you would probably want a full-bodied fragrance, say a spicy scent such as Shalimar, Opium or Cartier, or scents with a warm wooded aroma, perhaps Paloma Picasso. Why? When it's cold outside, our bodies do not give off as much energy, therefore a light floral fragrance might prove too fleeting. Unless, of course, that is the effect you want. Your choice in fragrance, like your choice in wine, should always be in sync with your personal preference.

Let's continue the story. Imagine early the next morning you board a plane for Acapulco for your winter vacation. When you arrive, it's nearly ninety degrees and humidity is high. At lunch you opt for a light salad and a delicate chilled white wine, or maybe clear sparkling water. It's a warm, sunny day and you're perspiring lightly or, as some might say, glowing. What fragrance should you wear? The full-bodied scent from last night might overwhelm you, so you choose a light, ethereal perfume instead. Something floral, fresh or fruity. You're glad you packed Chanel's Cristalle, Anaïs Anaïs and Nicole Miller. Perhaps a light veil of body lotion would suffice, or a dusting of powder. That evening, after an afternoon in the sun, you might smooth a glistening emollient body creme over your tender new tan, perhaps a scented creme like Pheromone or Lauren. Then it's back to the beach, to sip a chilled Piña Colada and watch the sun slip sienna toward the horizon.

These vignettes show how you can apply your soon-to-be-acquired knowledge of perfumery in everyday life to select just the right scents, prompting people to remark, "My, you smell wonderful!" The more than 350 Fragrance Profiles in Part 2 will give you the information you need for your experiments, plus stories about the history of some fragrances and the famous people who have worn them. Most of all, enjoy the discovery of the world's most elegant, romantic and sensual scents.

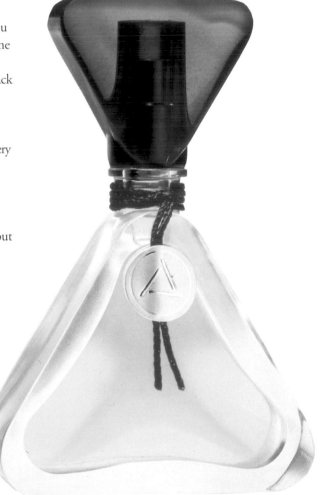

Liz Claiborne

Fashionable Scents of the Times

*Perfume is the unseen but unforgettable
and ultimate fashion accessory.
It heralds a woman's arrival and
prolongs her departure.*

Gabrielle "Coco" Chanel

Perfume reflects the period in which it
is created, like any work of art, literature or
fashion. From ancient times through today,
fragrance has mirrored the mood of the day.
Historical records show that the Greeks,
Romans, Egyptians, Arabs, Persians and Asians
produced scents for bathing, religious rituals,
banquets, entertaining and medicinal purposes.

Modern perfumery began in the seventeenth
century in the French town of Grasse, where
glovemakers used essences from the region's
flowers and plants to scent gloves. At that time,
leather was cured in a solution that left it with
an unsavory smell. Perfume was used to mask
this unpleasant odor, and scented gloves soon
became the rage.

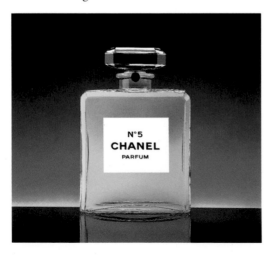

The eighteenth and nineteenth centuries
saw expanded fragrance usage. Lavender, violet
and rose were the lightly scented favorites of the
day. Empress Josephine loved rose water, while
Marie Antoinette went to her scaffold death
with two vials of Houbigant perfume ensconced
in her bosom for courage. Men and women
wore similar fragrances. It was the marketing-
savvy merchants of the twentieth century who
began to promote fragrances specifically
designed for each sex.

The early twentieth century saw rapid
technological advances, winds of social change,
daring new fashions. Heretofore scandalous
multi-floral scents became popular, as did spicy
Oriental blends. In the twenties and thirties
chemists experimented with new formulas,
using synthetic ingredients to create classic
scents that are still with us. The mood was
expansive: Joy, introduced as the costliest
perfume in the world, was snapped up by
Woolworth heiress Barbara Hutton, actresses
Mary Pickford and Constance Bennett, and
thousands of others. Couturiers branded
perfume with their own labels: Coco Chanel,
Paul Poiret, Jeanne Lanvin, Jean Patou, Charles
Worth. Dionne Warwick explains the success
of designer label perfumes: "Every woman
can't afford a designer dress, but she can wear
an original fragrance."

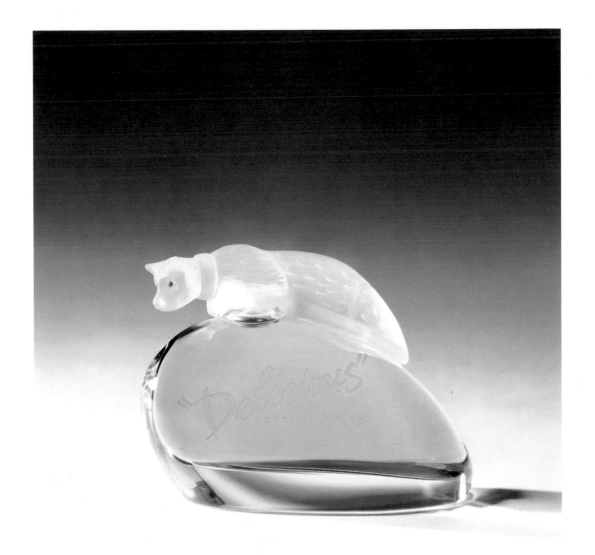

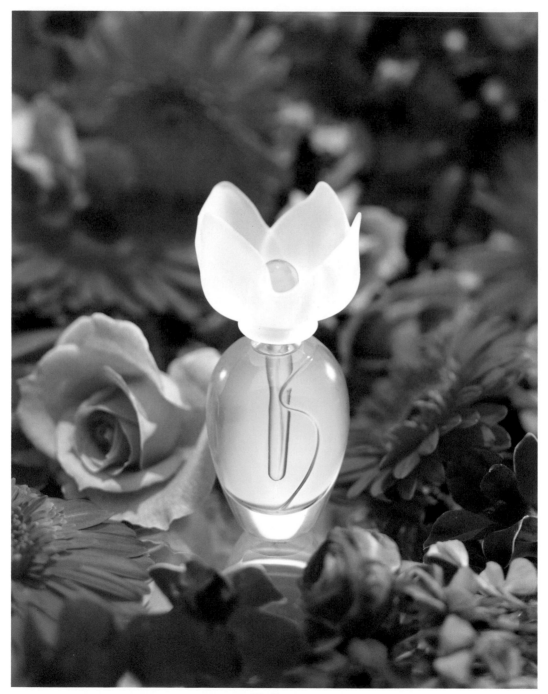

Chloé Narcisse

The late forties and fifties saw a return to feminine floral fragrances to complement the flowing skirts and tiny waists of Christian Dior's New Look fashions. Estée Lauder sparked demand in the United States for everyday perfume when she launched Youth Dew in 1953, a striking Oriental fragrance praised by Gloria Swanson, Joan Crawford, Dolores Del Rio and the Duchess of Windsor. Youth Dew's blockbuster appeal didn't go unnoticed by the large cosmetic and fragrance companies. The ensuing decades saw larger budgets, mega-launches and more designer imprints than ever.

The sixties and seventies were marked by the sexual revolution, civil rights and the women's movement. Fragrance recorded this with bold new scents laden with musk and patchouli. The greed-is-good eighties traded on glitz, intrigue, sex and money with fragrance hits like Obsession, Poison and Opium—distinctive, heady scents with rediscovered Oriental essences. And the designer race was heated. Not only were couture names recognizable and marketable, but designers wanted a piece of the dream, too. "The dream of any design house is to have its own proper fragrance," says Carla Fendi, "because when a woman gets dressed, the final touch is her fragrance." Calvin Klein, Bob Mackie and Gucci entered the fray along with Fendi.

The nineties are a back-to-basics, return-to-values time, and softer subtle scents are back in vogue. Fragrances with names like Realities, Delicious and ...with Love sum up the new attitude. Nineties scents are fresh, light and innocent, natural, fruity and herbal, but change is already is in the air for the coming century.

Before we go on, let's back up a bit and see where these fabulous fragrances come from.

Ingredients: The Building Blocks of Perfumery

The flowers regretfully shed tears of sweet perfume, as they would a treasured secret.

Charles Baudelaire

Fragrances are created from essential oils present in plants, flowers, fruits, bark, roots and animal secretions. And what precious, pricey substances they are! In Grasse, France, the center of the perfume industry, workers rise early to pick jasmine before dawn. When the sun peeks over the horizon, the flower loses twenty percent of its aroma. A skilled harvester can pick about a pound of flowers in forty-five minutes, or five thousand tiny blossoms. But only a few drops of essence will emerge after processing. Eight hundred pounds of jasmine flowers, or four million flowers, yields just one pound of concentrated oil. And the price for these essences? One pound of this oil, called jasmine absolute, will fetch $10,000 to $20,000, depending on quality, while rose absolute can cost as much as $6,000 per pound.

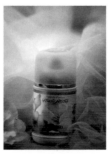

Anaïs-Anaïs

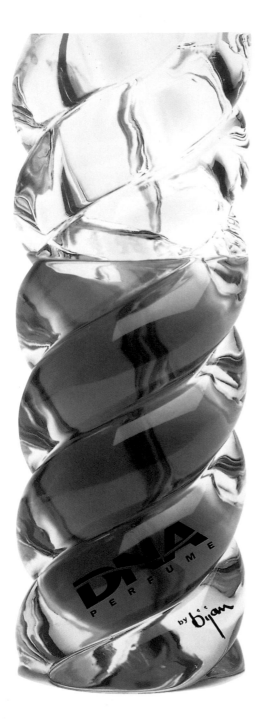

There's more. Indian sandalwood must mature for thirty to fifty years before harvest. Three thousand pounds of bergamot fruit from Calabria, Italy, will yield just two pounds of essence. Now consider that many perfumes have hundreds of different essential oils, and you will realize the precious artistry and gifts of nature that go into each bottle.

Keeping a fragrance unchanged over time is a challenge for art and science. For example, the scent of jasmine differs from field to field and year to year, depending on climate, rainfall and soil conditions. The chemist must tweak the formula to compensate for changes in ingredients. But to preserve the original perfume formulas, the French have established a library at the Osmathèque near Versailles.

Natural essences are often blended with laboratory-created ingredients from natural or chemical compounds. A synthetic may be created in imitation of natural aromas or as an entirely new aroma. Synthetics are far from poor substitutes for nature; many are more tenacious and costly than natural ingredients. The aldehydes in Chanel No. 5 are a sparkling example. And whereas only a few hundred fragrances are available for perfumery from nature, synthetic fragrances give the perfumer thousands. The combinations available today to the perfumer are virtually unlimited.

When is a rose not a rose? When the perfumer blends several components to give the impression of a rose. It is the essential oil or a combination of oils that evokes an aroma—be it woodsy, spicy, floral or something else.

A floral perfume may contain rose, violet or sandalwood. Or it may not, perhaps having been created by a combination of natural or synthetic materials that evoke such an aroma. This is how perfumers re-create the scent of the stubborn violet, which jealously refuses to yield its floral essence. The perfumer uses orris root, similar in fragrance to violet. Apricot is another example. Also re-created synthetically is musk, whose source in nature is the male musk deer.

For more guidance on specific ingredients, turn to the back of this book, where you'll find a list of Commonly Used Ingredients in Perfumery. For the unusual component not listed, turn to a dictionary or encyclopedia for more information.

Now we come to the next step: The assembly of ingredients into a perfume is called its "composition."

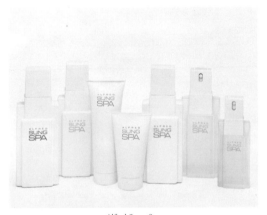

Alfred Sung Spa

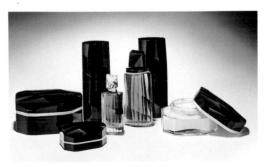

Mackie, Bob Mackie

Composition: Notable Notes

As in music, a fragrance is composed of notes, which can follow each other or overlap. Most fragrances pass through three phases when used, commonly structured this way:

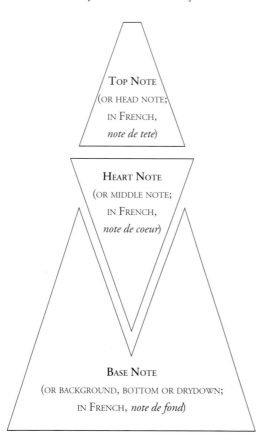

TOP NOTE
(OR HEAD NOTE;
IN FRENCH,
note de tete)

HEART NOTE
(OR MIDDLE NOTE;
IN FRENCH,
note de coeur)

BASE NOTE
(OR BACKGROUND, BOTTOM OR DRYDOWN;
IN FRENCH, *note de fond*)

The journey of a sensory experience begins in the bottle, where the first whiff is detected. The scent changes when applied to the skin, and it is different still an hour later.

The use of musical terms is no accident. In the nineteenth century, a French master perfumer devised a system whereby each essence was assigned a note based on a tonal scale spanning six and a half octaves. The term "note" can refer to a single ingredient, such as rose or sandalwood, or to the phase, as in top note.

The top note is the initial impression of the scent on the skin and is designed to be fleeting and volatile. It lasts less than a minute. As the fragrance interacts with skin chemistry, the next discernable aroma is the heart note. Several minutes later, the final or base note becomes evident. The base note is enhanced by fixatives, which give the fragrance stability and staying power. Only when the base note emerges will the true personality of the perfume reveal itself, as the scent notes blend with your personal chemistry.

Components are arranged according to their volatility, or how quickly they disperse into the air. Light, fresh ones are usually found in the top note—citrus, greens, aldehydes and delicate florals. The heart note contains the mid-range—rich florals—while warm woods and fixatives of a high molecular weight are placed in the background or base—sandalwood, vanilla, musk, vetiver, cedar, balsam, olibanum, incense and benzoin.

Although perfumes are designed in three phases—the top, heart and base—a common thread should run through the composition. Well-blended perfumes glide from one phase to the next with similar elements, rather than

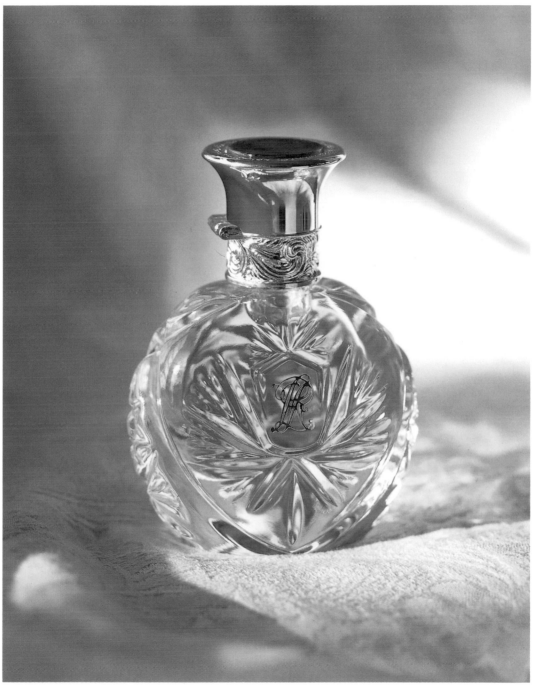

Safari

29

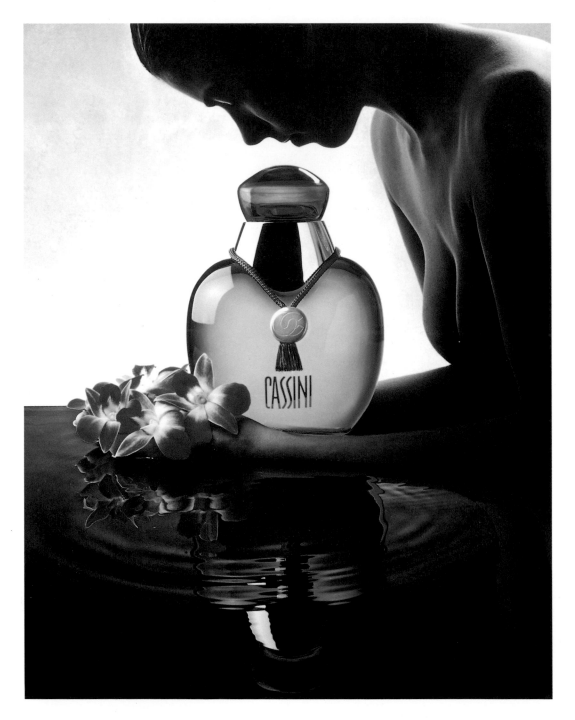

having three distinct phases. Think of a symphony with its highs and lows, quick and leisurely movements, but always with repetition of a theme.

The various phases occur because ingredients evaporate, or dry down, at different speeds as the alcohol in the perfume evaporates. Fruits, citrus and greens often dissipate quickly. Therefore crisp citrus is refreshing and invigorating, ideal for use in brisk top notes and cologne splashes. Animal fixatives are long-lasting, so ambergris, musk and civet are usually placed in the base to extend the fragrance. When properly blended, these rather pungent animal essences add superb body.

Musk is particularly potent, as one French Emperor reportedly found out. Musk was favored by Empress Josephine, wife of Napoléon. Legend has it that when her husband divorced her in 1809 to marry Archduchess Marie Louise of Austria the next year, Josephine doused her apartments with musk in a fit of fury before leaving. Walls, upholstery, draperies —she lavished it in every room, for she wanted to leave an indelible imprint, to make her memory inescapable. She vowed that Napoléon would never forget her. Besides, she knew that Marie Louise abhorred the smell of musk and wore only light violet scents. No doubt Josephine had smelled violet on her husband's collar, and Marie Louise had detected musk. It is said the apartments smelled of musk for decades after the unhappy departure.

Now let's move from the deeply personal to the impersonal—how perfumers categorize fragrance.

Scent Types

To bring order to their fragrant pursuit, perfumers divide fragrances into basic categories, or scent types, based on the main theme of the scent. In this book, we use a standard industry system used by noted fragrance firms such as Haarmann & Reimer, as well as information contributed by fragrance companies for specific scents. The main women's categories are:

FLORAL   *CITRUS*

ORIENTAL   *FOUGÈRE*

CHYPRE   *GREEN*

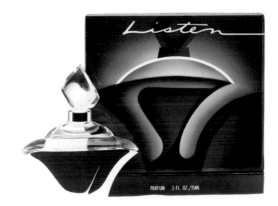

These categories are further divided to reflect variations on the main theme:

Floral   - Green
         - Fruity
         - Fresh
         - Aldehyde
         - Ambery
         - Oriental
Oriental - Ambery
         - Spicy
Chypre   - Fruity
         - Floral-Animalic
         - Floral
         - Fresh
         - Green
Citrus
Fougère
Green

Many of the citrus fragrances are a light eau de cologne that can be worn by women and men. In the Profiles, you'll also see many category blends, such as Floral - Oriental. Note that these categories reflect the dominant theme, but other elements are also present, for example, a hint of greenery in a spicy Oriental blend. And fragrances are usually balanced with ingredients that serve to stabilize or extend the scent, such as woods or mosses, even though the main theme might be a floral or citrus.

(Note: Because of the chemistry involved, the dominant note impressions, not always actual ingredients, are recorded under the Composition heading in the Fragrance Profiles in Part 2.)

Now let's look more closely at each scent type:

FLORAL

The largest number of fragrances fall into the floral category. Some are single floral fragrances, although most are richer multi-floral bouquets with ingredients such as jasmine, rose, gardenia, ylang-ylang, hyacinth, honeysuckle, tuberose, lilac, lily of the valley, narcissus, violet, carnation, lavender, orange blossom and magnolia. These bouquets range from medium strength to high intensity. A few popular floral compositions are Chloé, Delicious, Beautiful, Jardins de Bagatelle, Joy, Sublime, Paris, White Shoulders, Vivid, Carolina Herrera, Alexander Julian's Womenswear, Fred Hayman's Touch and 273, and Elizabeth Taylor's White Diamonds.

Floral - Green

This version of the floral theme has green notes that conjure up images of freshly mown lawns and spring meadows. Green notes can be described as vigorous, crisp and refreshing, and are made of grasses, leaves, lavender, basil, chamomile, hyacinth and galbanum. Chanel No. 19, Safari, Alfred Sung, Jessica McClintock, Vent Vert and Cabotine are green floral blends.

Floral - Fruity

The fruity accented floral theme is known for its succulent radiance and ethereal lightness. Pineapple, mandarin, peach, plum, raspberry, apricot and apple are often used for their casual freshness. Enjoying a budding demand in the nineties are fruity floral scents such as Giò, Il Bacio, Tribù, Calyx, Nicole Miller, Lauren, Liz Claiborne, Romeo Gigli, Design, Listen, Escape, Amarige and Senso.

Floral - Fresh

Delicate spring-like freshness characterizes the fresh floral category. Lightness is achieved by the fleeting qualities of florals such as orange blossom and lily of the valley. Citrus fruits of lemon and bergamot are often used to lighten the floral bouquet, while a subtle, powdery trail is another hallmark of this category. Favorite fragrances that fall into this dimension are Anaïs Anaïs, Moods, Destiny, Amour Amour and EarthSource Rainswept Jasmine.

Floral - Aldehyde

Synthetically created aldehydes were popularized in the 1920s, when they were first used in perfumery. Aldehydes represent entirely new fragrances not found in nature and can add unusual characteristics—sparkling, sharp, elegant or powerful. Chanel No. 5 is perhaps the most famous floral aldehyde and is joined by Arpège, Calandre, First, Red, Nahema, Liu, Bois des Îles, Calèche and White Linen. One of our favorite stories about a floral aldehyde perfume is from Marilyn Monroe: When the press once asked what she wore to bed, she smiled and answered simply, "Chanel No. 5."

Floral - Ambery

These are fragrances whose ambery quality adds a heavy, warm sweetness to rich floral compositions. Many fragrances in this category have Oriental ingredients such as vanilla, balsam and spice, and they sometimes overlap with Floral Orientals, a category that we have separated. Bijan's DNA, Tiffany, L'Heure Blue, Oscar de la Renta, and Caesars Woman are well-known floral ambery fragrances.

Floral - Oriental

Floral Oriental is a blend of exotic floral essences and warm Oriental ingredients of spice, balsam or resin. A semi-Oriental is softer, subtle. A fragrance theme that has many entrants, floral Orientals include Coco, Bijan, Venezia, Moschino, Escada, Vanderbilt, Chloé Narcisse, Realities, Jil Sander No. 4, Dolce & Gabbana, Bob Mackie, Alfred Sung E.N.C.O.R.E., Diamonds and Rubies, Samsara and ...with Love. Trésor and Boucheron are floral semi-Orientals.

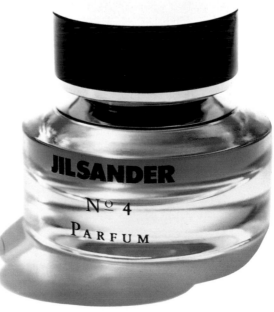

ORIENTAL

Oriental fragrances are those that conjure up images of the Far East, of spices and musk and resins, of exotic flowers and sweet warm balsam. Oriental blends are actually more popular in the Western Hemisphere, owing to their highly fragrant nature. Oriental fragrances are the heaviest fragrance category, warm and sultry; they are ideal for cool weather and evening wear. Guerlain's Shalimar is a particularly memorable Oriental and was one of the first created. Angel, Realm, Nuit de Noël, Coquette and Royal Secret are among other Oriental favorites. Colors de Benetton is a softer version; a semi-Oriental.

Oriental - Ambery

This fragrance subset puts a citrusy culinary spin on the Oriental theme by blending fresh citrus with amber and vanilla. Sounds almost good enough to eat, although we certainly don't recommend it—even though Scarlett O'Hara gargled perfume to cover the alcohol on her breath in *Gone with the Wind.* For sought-after scents in this category, think of Roma, Obsession, Must de Cartier, Ciara, Dionne, Habanita and Normandie.

Oriental - Spicy

A high dose of spice distinguishes this version of the Oriental theme. This type of fragrance may seem familiar to most people because these spices are used in cooking—cinnamon, nutmeg, vanilla, pepper, clove, ginger, coriander, cardamom. Spicy florals such as carnation and lavender may round out the formulas, which are often backed up with musk and dry woods. These spice blends are found in KL, Cinnabar, Opium, Parfum Sacré, Tianne and Teatro alla Scala. Notable fragrances that are an Oriental ambery-spicy blend are Guerlain's Vol de Nuit, Bal à Versailles and Youth Dew, said to be one of Madonna's favorites.

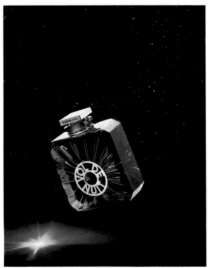

Vol de Nuit

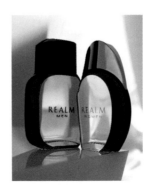

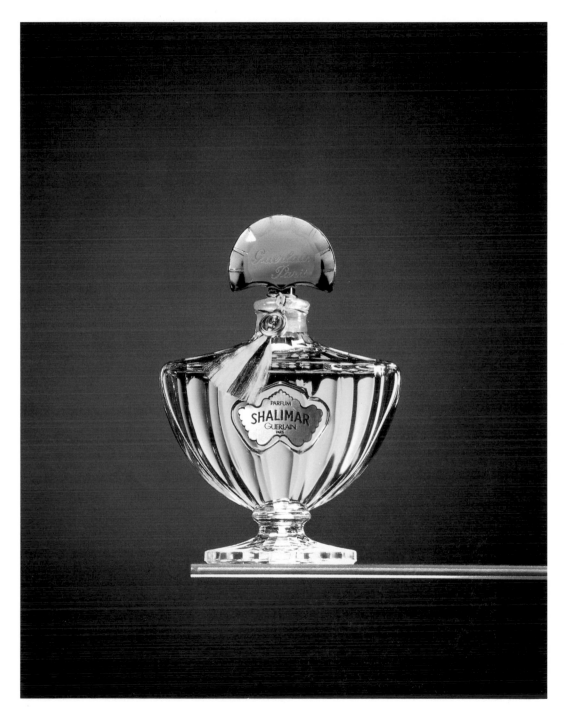

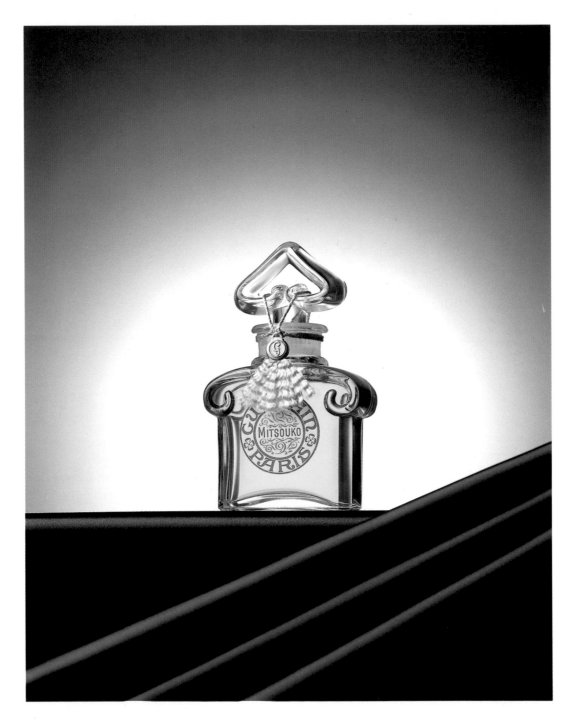

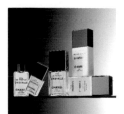

Cristalle

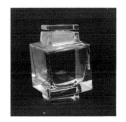

V'E' Versace

CHYPRE

The chypre theme is often described as woodsy-mossy. The word "chypre" can be traced to François Coty, who created a perfume to mirror the aromas he encountered on the Mediterranean island of Cyprus. He called his fragrance Chypre, which is French for Cyprus. In English, pronounce it "sheep-ra," with a French accent. Although Coty's Chypre perfume is no longer being made, the name stuck and today is applied to all compositions exhibiting the qualities of the original. As with other fragrance themes, there are several subsets, but the main concept is a marriage of fresh citrus and oakmoss. An inedible fruit called bergamot is preferred for its crisp nature, which blends well with the earthy oakmoss and the often-used patchouli. The result is natural and foresty, soft, sweet and warm. Enigma and Feminité du Bois are two examples of this category.

Chypre - Fruity

A heavier variation is the fruity theme, which imparts a mellow warmth to the classic chypre composition realized through the addition of peach. Well-known interpretations include Mitsouko, Femme, Gem, Cocktail and Colony.

Chypre - Floral - Animalic

The fullest interpretation of the chypre theme is achieved through the blending of florals and animal essences. Animal notes include secretions from civet cats and musk deer, whale ambergris and beaver castoreum—though today they are generally synthetic reproductions. Not particularly appealing on their own, these components add magnificent warmth, tenacity and roundness to compositions when properly used. To see for yourself, try a few: Ysatis, Miss Dior, Cuir de Russie, Givenchy III, Moments and Jolie Madame.

Chypre - Floral

A lighter version of the above classification is the chypre floral, made by downplaying the animal notes and moving rich florals to center stage, still supported with zesty citrus, green oakmoss and woody patchouli. Rose and gardenia are the favored florals. To experience this production, look for Paloma Picasso, V'E Versace, Diva, Chant d'Arômes, Coriandre and Aromatics Elixir. Cassini is a fine example of a chypre floral-fruity blend.

Chypre - Fresh

This lighter variation of the chypre theme highlights the freshness of citrus. Favorite fragrances here are Cristalle, 4711 Eau de Cologne, Eau d'Hadrien and Eau de Rochas.

Chypre - Green

As the lightest of the chypre concept, the green theme is made with nature-inspired additions of grasses, leaves, lavender, basil, chamomile, hyacinth and galbanum. Coniferous notes may include pine, juniper and fir, while deeper herbal notes are achieved with sage and rosemary. The result is sporty and casual, with a stronger forest aroma than detected in the Floral Green theme. Wrappings, Private Collection and Aliage are green chypre arrangements.

CITRUS

Usually thought of as a male fragrance category, the citrus theme is increasingly popular among women. The citrus concept is one of the oldest and dates back to the early eau de cologne. Tangerine, lime, lemon, bergamot and mandarin are among citrus fruits commonly used—often called hesperides. Variations are realized by adding florals, greens and woods. Generally described as refreshing and exhilarating, citrus compositions can be used by women or men. Many women like the natural, casual appeal of scents such as Eau de Patou, Eau de Guerlain, Eau de Cologne Impériale, Eau de Cologne du Coq and Eau de Cologne Hermès.

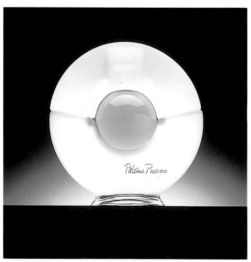

Paloma Picasso

FOUGÈRE

Another fragrance concept is the fougère theme, which means "fern" in French. Pronounce it "foozh-air." It is a well-balanced interpretation of the fresh green fern, with dominant notes of lavender, citrus, herbs and oakmoss. Florals, woods and animal notes may round out the fresh symphony. Today fougère notes are more often used in men's fragrances. Guerlain's Jicky is an enduring example of the fougère theme, a scent that can be worn by women and men.

GREEN

Finally, some fragrances have dominant green notes, like vigorous pine and juniper, dry herbs such as sage and rosemary, and fresh crisp notes from grasses, leaves, lavender, basil, chamomile, hyacinth and galbanum. Refreshing sporty scents, these are well-illustrated by the fashionable Pheromone, Reverie and Sung Spa.

So as you select fragrances, consider the overall scent type or category that they fall into as well as notes. In Part 2, each Profile will list first the Scent Type—Floral, Oriental, Citrus, etc.—followed by the Composition notes or ingredients, divided into top, heart and base. Before long you'll be able to detect the differences on your own.

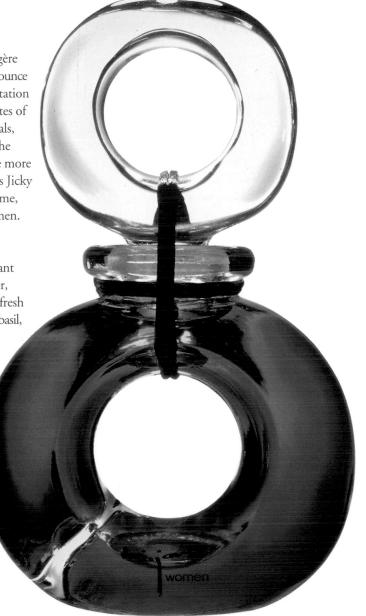

Bijan

How to Let Fragrance Work Best For You

Perfume, like glamour, is intangible and magnetic. Now that we've trekked through the jungle of scent types and composition, we're ready to explore the usage of fragrance. Let's look first at skin chemistry, product types and shopping for fragrance, then learn the concepts of layering and wardrobing.

Just as a symphony sounds different when performed by different musicians, a fragrance differs when worn by different individuals.

Why? The answer is varying skin chemistry. Acid balance, diet, medication, skin oil, pigmentation, mood and environmental factors influence how a fragrance develops on the skin as well as its staying power. You may notice a change in the way your favorite fragrances smell on you if you've changed your diet, if you've moved to a new climate, if you're taking new medication, or if you're under more stress than usual. Or perhaps you're so accustomed to your regular perfume that you've simply can't detect it when you wear it. If so, ask friends before you put more on—it may already be strong enough. It might also be time to experiment with new fragrances.

People with a higher proportion of body fat retain scent longer and may find fragrance to be stronger or sharper on their skin than on a friend's. Oily or darker skin also retains scent longer than dry or paler skin. You may find that your fragrance is disappearing if your skin is dry, or if you're on a low-fat diet with a strenuous exercise regime, or if you live in a cold, harsh climate. What to do? Try using a full-strength perfume, along with bath oils, lotions and cremes in the same scent family to extend your fragrance. On the other hand, if your skin is dark or oily, or the temperature is rising, you may want to use less fragrance or switch to a lighter scent, especially for daytime or professional wear. Look for fresh or fruity florals, citrus, or green scents. Try an eau de toilette, eau de cologne, or splash.

It is wise to use lighter scents in the daytime if you work in a crowded office. Reserve your heady, sensual perfumes for the evening hours when the temperature drops—or for maximum impact with that special someone. The general rule is the earlier the hour, the lighter the scent.

Seasons also matter. Many women like a heady floral, heavy spice, or sensual Oriental fragrance in the winter. In the heat of the summer they select a lighter floral, citrus or green in the form of a soft perfume, a light cologne, or an eau de toilette. This is because more fragrance is emanated as the body perspires.

Elizabeth Taylor's Diamonds and Sapphires, Diamonds and Rubies, Diamonds and Emeralds.

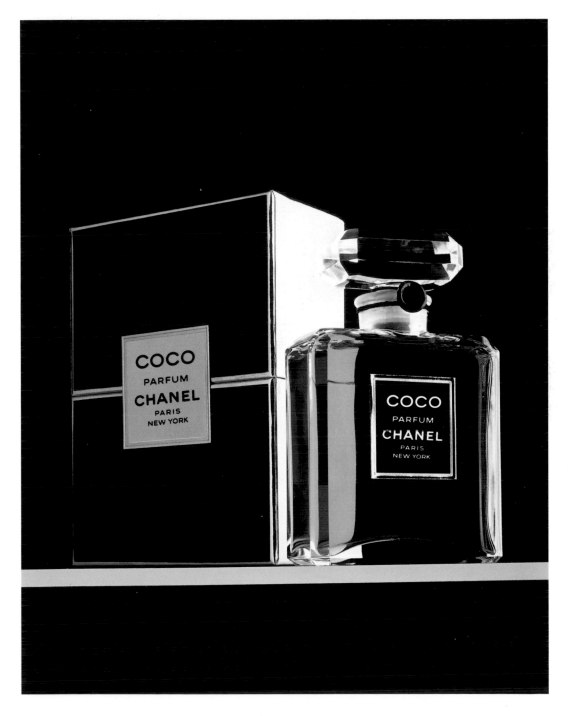

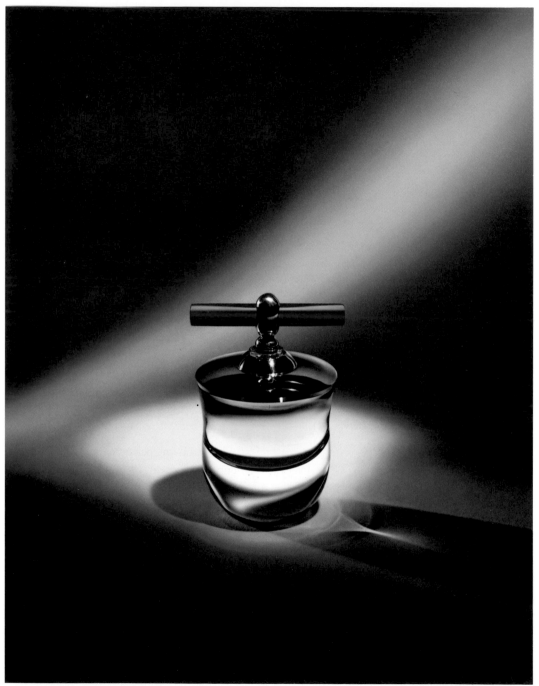

Vivid

42

Fragrance Strengths and Products

The next step is to understand the strength of fragrances available. Perfume is the most intense form of fragrance, followed by eau de parfum, eau de toilette and cologne. Some fragrance companies market a light perfume, which is midway between perfume and eau de parfum. Naturally, the more fragrance oils, or compound, used in a formula, the longer the fragrance will last, and the higher the retail price will be.

Fragrance Strengths

	Percentage of Fragrance Compound
Perfume (also Parfum, Extrait)	15% to 30%
Eau de Parfum	8% to 15%
Eau de Toilette	4% to 8%
Eau de Cologne	2% to 5%
Splash Cologne	1% to 3%

Source: The Fragrance Foundation

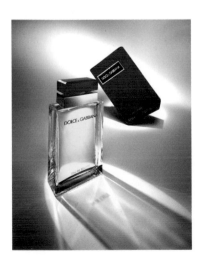

Eau de toilette and cologne are designed to be used lavishly over the entire body and usually come in large spray or splash bottles. Eau de parfum is a more concentrated version with longer staying power—fine for cooler weather or dryer skin. It is usually available in a spray or splash and is designed to be used with only a little less restraint than an eau de toilette, highlighting the pulse points.

Perfume is generally packaged in a flacon, or perfume bottle with a tight-fitting cap, to guard against evaporation of the rich, precious compound. Use perfume for maximum impact and longer enjoyment. While the initial investment for perfume is higher than for a less concentrated form of the scent, perfume will last longer on your body and remain truer to the scent. The ounce of perfume, used properly, will far outlast the large size eau de toilette that demands frequent application. In France, perfume outsells the less concentrated forms, for French women know and value the concentrated perfumes. But many women prefer less concentrated sprays that they can use lavishly. It's a matter of personal choice.

When buying perfume, purchase only the amount you'll use quickly, because fragrance companies say perfume has a shelf life of six to eighteen months after opening, or up to three years if sealed. But test it; we've had fragrance last even longer. Perhaps a quarter- or half-ounce is a better buy if you use it slowly. Once you open a bottle of perfume, enjoy it—don't save it for special occasions. If you find your fragrance looking thicker or darker, it is spoiling and the scent may be altered. Use it or lose it!

Different fragrance strengths in a fragrance line—perfume, eau de toilette, eau de parfum—are usually formulated to give a similar impression, but since they are unique compositions, they will differ to a degree. For example, an eau de toilette may have a burst of scent and dry down quickly, while a perfume evolves slowly and lasts longer. Each is unique; experiment to find which product or combination suits you best.

Spray perfume on pulse points to warm and disperse the fragrance most effectively—behind the ears, on the neck, between the breasts, at the bend in elbows and knees...even at the ankles, for fragrance rises. Coco Chanel said, "Perfume should be sprayed wherever you expect to be kissed."

A spray is better than dabbing perfume with fingers, because your skin oils can enter the bottle and cause the perfume to spoil faster. Spraying fragrance will also result in a finer, more even application. Look for elegant atomizers in the perfume departments to cradle your favorite perfumes.

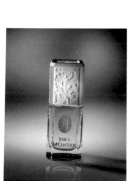

Jessica McClintock

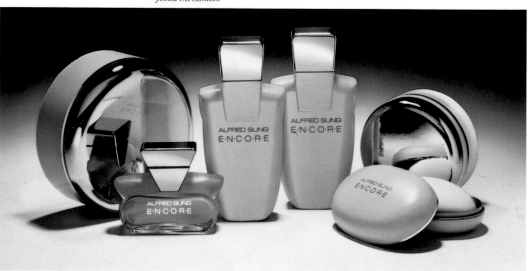

Another fragrance-saving tip: Store your fragrance bottles away from direct sunlight and extreme heat. Even though the bottles may be dark colored, the sun can damage delicate fragrance oils. Some women even store their fine perfume in the refrigerator. But be careful, or the butter may begin to take on the scent of your favorite perfume—use a plastic bag!

Bath oil can be used in a similar fashion to perfume, as well as in the bath. It is usually less costly, and is oil-based rather than alcohol-based. Estée Lauder's Youth Dew is a popular fragrance that was introduced as a bath oil and fragrance. But, as with all fragrance, take care to keep the oil away from your clothing as it may stain.

Many fragrance lines contain a light lotion or moisturizing fluid. For maximum hydrating treatment and a higher concentration of perfume oil, try the rich emollient cremes, usually packaged in jars. These are best applied to slightly damp skin. Top with dusting powder or talc to set the fragrance, just as powder applied to the face sets the foundation base. The lotion and powder alone, sans liquid fragrance, may suffice for daytime or hot climate wear.

Scented bath products are a wonderful addition to the bathing ritual. But remember, a deodorant soap is designed to kill odors, and unfortunately it cannot distinguish a fine fragrance. Even though the deodorant soap is washed off, its lingering residue continues to battle odors for hours, including that of your favorite perfume or body lotion. Solve this by using a mild, unscented soap, or a soap from your fragrance wardrobe.

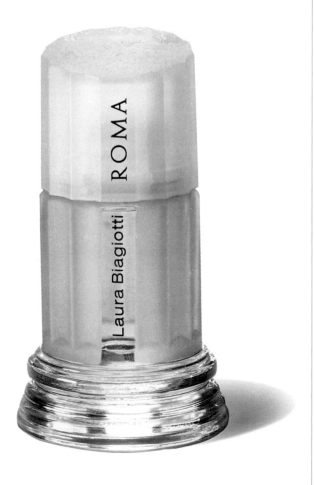

Layering Fragrance

Scent staying power can be increased by layering several forms of the fragrance together. For example, you may begin with the scented soap or bath oil, follow with scented body lotion or creme, dust with scented powder, and for the finale, indulge in a luxurious spritz of the liquid aroma.

Layering results in a more even application of the fragrance, clothing the wearer from head to toe in a cloud of fragrance like an aura. It is perfect for women with dry skin who have trouble retaining fragrance, or in cool climates. And remember to carry a purse-size flacon of the perfume to touch up later in the day.

Some women create their own fragrances by combining scents. One actress we know—Josette Banzet from *The Other Side of Midnight* and *Rich Man, Poor Man*—layers the body creme from one scent with the perfume of another. Her favorite combination is Shalimar and Must de Cartier. Both are Oriental fragrances, and the result is delightful. This can work well with fragrances of the same scent type, but use caution when mixing fragrances from different fragrance families. The key is to try it at home first.

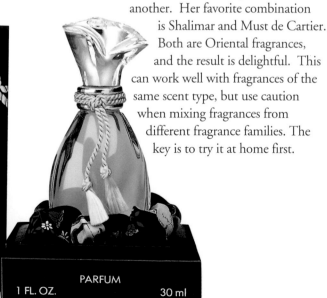

PARFUM

1 FL. OZ.   30 ml

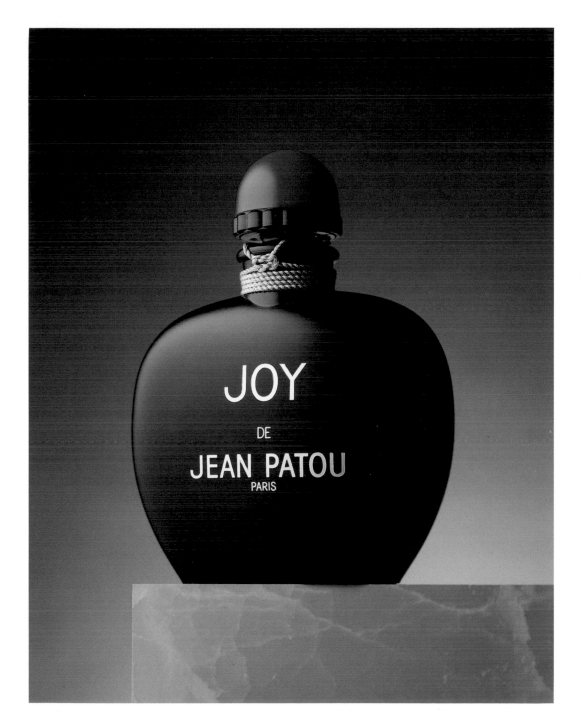

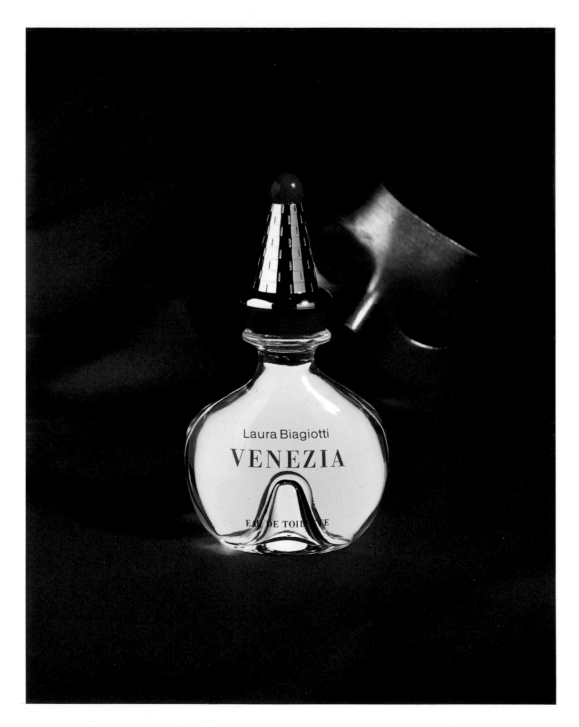

Shopping for Fragrance

We are often asked, "How do I find a perfume that is right for me?" As we've said, experiment! When you shop for scents, limit your trial to three or four fragrances or you'll overwhelm your sensory perception. Take home samples when they are available, so you can have more than one trial run in a variety of settings.

Try this: Sample scents in certain places on your skin, say one fragrance on the back of your right hand and another on the inside of your right forearm, then apply two others to the left side. Jot down what you've tried in each spot, so you'll remember what you've applied where as the scents develop on your skin.

Sniff periodically over an hour or two, away from the fragrance-laden cosmetic department. Notice how each fragrance develops differently on your skin as it mingles with your skin chemistry. Also note any allergic reactions.

When you're shopping you're sure to encounter a myriad of sexy, glamorous ads. While you shouldn't base your perfume purchase on the name or ten million dollar-plus advertising campaign, elements are often chosen to reflect the fragrance's personality. Fashion and change are fun, but don't be swayed—let your nose be the ultimate authority, regardless of the trend. Select the scents that are best on you and most appropriate for the occasion.

Perhaps you once tried a fragrance, but now you can't find it in a store near you. Don't worry. Most fragrances profiled in this book are carried in fine department stores, but if you have trouble locating a scent, turn to our Buyer's Guide for names and telephone numbers of distributors. Most will refer you to a store in your area,

though some might ship directly to you. Duty free shops and specialty perfume stores are also excellent at locating particular scents, even if they don't normally stock them. And don't forget, when outside the country, check the local perfumeries.

If you have to ask the price—and don't we all today?—we're here to help. Here's a quote we thought appropriate from John Dryden, a seventeenth-century English dramatist:

The sweetest essences are always contained in the smallest glasses.

Since price fluctuates, we've given a price range for each fragrance, based on the per-ounce price for perfume. Of course, less concentrated versions are less costly.

At the time of writing, perfumes fell into the following price ranges:

1 ounce Perfume

	(from:)
Mid-range	$125
High range	$200
Top range	$300

All prices are in U.S. Dollars.

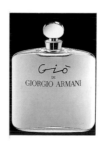

Some fragrances are not produced in a perfume version. We've classified those according to their range in the fragrance strength produced.

In this book, we selected the prestige perfumes found in fine department stores and perfumeries. You may have less expensive favorites, but with more than eight hundred fragrances on the market, we had to make the cut somewhere! We handpicked more than three hundred fifty favorite prestige fragrances for the Profiles, and included sixty more as Honorable Mentions. That should keep you busy for some time...it certainly did us.

You may also find fragrances that have been discontinued. The world changes so fast around us—classic scents such as Arpège are often revived; distributors drop a fragrance from their stable, only to have it picked up by another distributor later; some fragrances live on in other countries; others cease production but the fragrance remains on the retail shelf for some time. We included old favorites so that you can compare fragrances and perhaps find a suitable replacement.

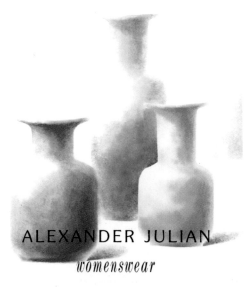

ALEXANDER JULIAN

womenswear

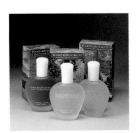

EarthSource Collection

Fragrance Wardrobing

A fragrance wardrobe is like a clothing wardrobe. You'll want fragrances for different occasions, moods, hours and climates. Some people wear just one fragrance, like the Balanchine and Russian ballerinas who were assigned one perfume to wear at all times (and intensely on stage). Most people, however, will enjoy the diversity of wardrobing. Why, even the French King Louis XV was a devout believer in fragrance wardrobes—he insisted his court wear a different perfume for every day of the week.

The Fragrance Foundation, an industry association, suggests a minimum of four scent types to start a wardrobe: a floral, an Oriental, a chypre or woodsy-mossy and a green. These will carry you through various climates and occasions, and you can enhance your wardrobe from there. To help in your selections, flip to the back of this book to find the Profile Fragrances by Scent Type.

The Memorable Impact of Fragrance

It is impossible to explore fragrances without also examining how fragrance benefits us. Scientists are discovering that the sense of smell may be the strongest sense we have. Perhaps Oliver Wendell Holmes said it best:

Memories, imagination, old sentiments and associations are more readily reached through the sense of smell than through any other channel.

Our sense of smell is an automatic memory trigger and is the most direct link to the brain and limbic system, where memories are stored. Every time we inhale, our brains register smells, consciously or unconsciously. Certain scents are stimulating, others are relaxing. Fragrance appeals to our basic instincts, and it is upon this appeal that the fragrance industry was built.

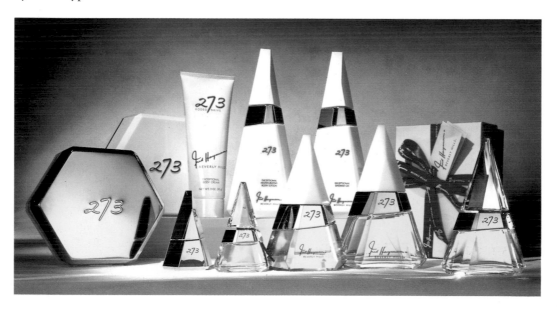

Neiman Marcus fragrance expert Bunni Nance says: "Many times, when a male customer encounters the scent of a perfume once worn by a loved one—mother, wife, girlfriend, grandmother—they are overwhelmed to tears. The memories flood back, and they simply must have that perfume again." Vivid memories —powerful feelings.

Aroma-Chology and Aromatherapy

He set himself to discover what there was in frankincense that made one mystical; and in ambergris that stirred one's passions; and in violets that woke the memory of dead romances; and in musk that troubled the brain; and in champak that stained the imagination.

Oscar Wilde

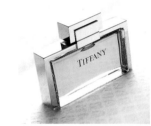

Our sense of smell is related to our sense of well-being. Two disciplines are dedicated to this truth, aromatherapy and aroma-chology. The noted industry association, the Olfactory Research Fund, defines aromatherapy as "the therapeutic use of pure essential oils and herbs, the result of which is described by proponents as 'healing, beautifying and soothing' the body and mind." Aromatherapy uses only pure, natural oils from plants and herbs. The term "aromatherapy" was coined in the 1930s, but this art has been practiced for 5,000 years. It uses only pure, natural essential oils.

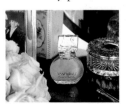

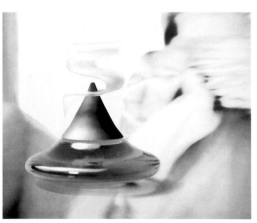

Romeo Gigli

Vanderbilt

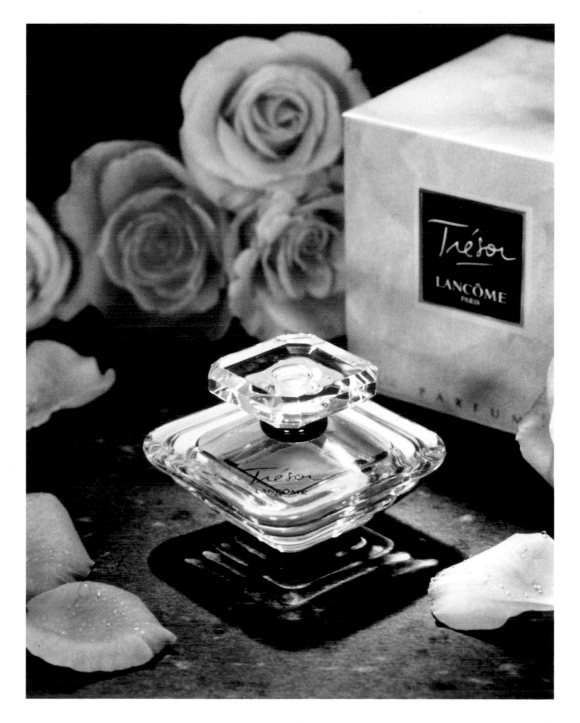

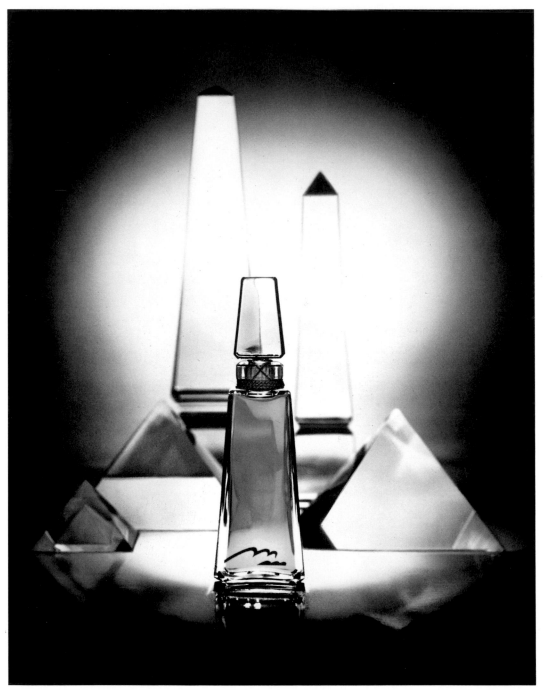

Pheromone

54

The Olfactory Research Fund defines aroma-chology as "a science developed by the Olfactory Research Fund, which is dedicated to the study of the inter-relationship of psychology and the latest in fragrance technology to transmit through odor a variety of specific feelings...relaxation, exhilaration, sensuality, happiness and achievement...directly to the pleasure center of the brain (the seat of emotions, memory, creativity and sensuality)."

Through tests, psychologists have found that peppermint and lily of the valley are stimulants and actually make students more alert during tests as well as increasing their scores. How much better? About 25% on average. Automobile drivers report a similar improvement in mental alertness when a peppermint air freshener is used.

Many Japanese firms spurt fragrance into the office air. During one test with keypunch operators, a company found a 21% error reduction with lavender, a 33% error drop with jasmine, and an astounding 54% error reduction with lemon. Plus, the operators said they felt better in the fragrant environment. On the other hand, psychologists have discovered that some odors are relaxants. For example, researchers at New York's Sloan-Kettering Cancer Institute have found that the scent of vanilla can relax patients undergoing magnetic resonance imaging (MRI).

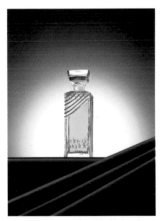

Jardins de Bagatelle

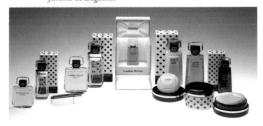

Carolina Herrera

Some other scents and their uses are:

Usage	Aroma	Usage	Aroma
Relieving Anxiety	*Cedarwood, basil, bergamot*	Relieving PMS	*Chamomile, galbanum, clary sage, neroli, tonka bean*
Relieving Depression	*Tuberose, fir, osmanthus, hyacinth, lily of the valley, bergamot, rose, neroli, ylang-ylang, nutmeg, basil, tonka bean, geranium*	Heightening Sensuality	*Hyacinth, musk, jasmine, rose, patchouli, civet, ambergris, clove, ginger, tuberose, sandalwood, ylang-ylang, mimosa, tagetes, neroli, vetiver, tonka bean*
Freshening Air	*Eucalyptus, cinnamon, clove, rosemary, thyme, lemon, bergamot, sage*	Stimulating	*Jasmine, lemon, peppermint, lily of the valley, osmanthus, hyacinth*
Encouraging Happiness	*Lily of the valley, tuberose, fir, osmanthus, hyacinth*	Reducing Stress	*Rose, tuberose, osmanthus, hyacinth, vetiver, lavender, galbanum, neroli*
Curing Insomnia	*Lavender, clary sage, chamomile, basil, vanilla, heliotropine, rose, sandalwood, tagetes*	Relaxing	*Chamomile, vanilla, apple spice, lavender, lily of the valley, tuberose, fir, hyacinth, geranium, orange, rose*
Invigorating	*Eucalyptus, pine*		
Improving Mental Efficiency	*Rose, basil, bergamot, lemon, cardamom, mint, grapefruit, pine, juniper*		

Sources: The Fragrance Foundation, Olfactory Research Fund, International Flavors and Fragrances, The Complete Aromatherapy Handbook

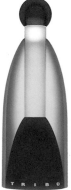

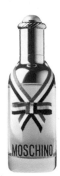

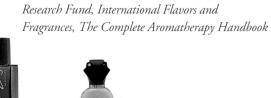

Design

Note that stimulation and relaxation are not mutually exclusive states. Some essences induce a state of calm vitality by reducing stress but increase energy and alertness.

Fragrance can be used to improve moods. A study by the world's largest fragrance manufacturer, International Flavors and Fragrances, found specific psychological effects from certain fragrances. For example, Douglas fir is relaxing, tuberose is relaxing and sensuous, and osmanthus is stimulating and encourages happiness. Hyacinth has a wealth of goodness; it promotes calm vitality through happiness, sensuality, stimulation and relaxation, while decreasing negative moods.

But wait, there's more. Dr. Susan Schiffman of Duke Medical Center and Hospital tested women and found that daily use of fragrance lifted their moods—even if they didn't particularly like the fragrance. Tension, anxiety, fatigue and inertia were dramatically reduced when the women liked the fragrance.

Can fragrance help to lose weight? Schiffman thinks so. Through studies, she found that overweight people want more intense and varied aromas from their food. They have a heightened sensory pleasure in eating. She believes weight loss can be aided by adding strong and varied flavors to a low-fat diet.

For centuries perfume has also been recognized for its aphrodisiac powers. Scents valued for their aphrodisiac qualities include jasmine, clove, ginger, violet and patchouli. Some people believe rose to be as powerful as a narcotic. Finally, ambergris, musk and civet are among the most sensually attractive essences.

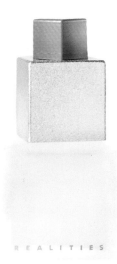

REALITIES

We recently asked, what does the future in fragrance hold? "In the future, people will be interested in fragrance plus its benefit," says Annette Green, head of The Fragrance Foundation headquartered in New York, an industry association. "Not only will they purchase fragrance for its aroma, but also for the extra benefits revealed by research in the new science of aroma-chology."

The trend in aroma-chology-inspired products has already begun. Fragrance and cosmetic companies like Origins and the Body Shop are riding high on the new wave of fragrance developments.

The Envelope, Please

As you read the Fragrance Profiles in Part 2, you will find references to The Fragrance Foundation, the nonprofit association of the fragrance industry. Each year the Foundation recognizes achievement in several categories at an awards ceremony. Incorporating the Foundation's initials, *Beauty Fashion* and *Cosmetic World* publisher John Ledes nicknamed the awards "FiFis." The FiFi Awards are considered the Oscar equivalent in the fragrance industry.

Let the Journey Begin

As you enter the world of fragrance, consider the exquisite words of Helen Keller, whose sense of smell was paramount:

Even as I think of smells,
my nose is full of scents
that start awake sweet memories
of summers gone
and ripening fields far away.

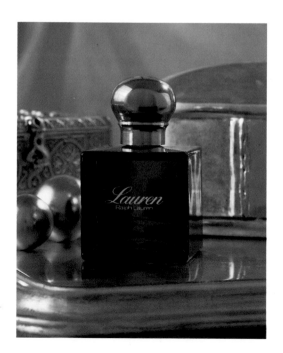

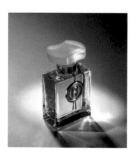

Fred Hayman's Touch

PART 2

ADORATION

Scent Type
  Floral
Composition
  Top Notes: *Freesia*
  Heart and Base Notes: *Apricot blossoms*

Famous Patrons
  Princess Diana of Wales
  Hillary Rodham Clinton

Adoration is a fresh, natural fragrance, resplendent with English freesia and sweet apricot. Fine fragrance purveyor William Owen III describes this scent as "cool and flirtatious, and when worn, the name happens." Perfect for warm weather, daytime, anytime. The effect is subtle, soft, sensuous sophistication, fit for royalty. In fact, English-born Owen created Adoration for Princess Diana.

Owen was born into a family of perfumers who have created memorable scents for European royalty for generations. Now residing in Palm Beach, Florida, Owen is a man of many passions, including antique perfume flacons, lavish millinery, vintage Rolls-Royces (including one from the Prince Aga Khan) and a dog named Bertie. His artistry in perfumes has long been recognized by a select group of women who discover his fragrances at the House of Isis in England, by appointment only, of course. Elsewhere, Owen scents can be found at exclusive department stores.

The natural fragrance is ensconced in glamorous packaging, designed by Owen and graced with his elegant drawings. The perfume is beautifully attired in cut-crystal bottles resting amidst silken French brocade. The perfume comes in two versions, one in a plain cut-crystal bottle, the other with sparkling pavé Swarovski crystals from Austria, set in 22-karat gold. The "totally jeweled" perfume flacons are to die for—dazzling purse-size containers you'll love using, drenched in crystals and accented with Swarovski "rubies."

The colognes and perfumes are priced for any budget, from a mere $10 for a half-dram of perfume to $1,000 for a 3.4-ounce jeweled "absolute essence." Definitely worth looking for.

Introduced   1991
Price   *Mid- to High range*

ALEXANDRA

Scent Type
  Semi-Oriental
Composition
  Top Notes: *Italian iris,*
  South African marigold
  Heart Notes: *French jasmine,*
  Moroccan rose, French jonquil
  Base Notes: *Indian sandalwood,*
  Singapore patchouli, Réunion Island vetiver

A classic semi-Oriental fragrance from Alexandra de Markoff, Alexandra is composed of rare essences from around the world.

If you haven't tried the Alexandra de Markoff cosmetic line lately, you're in for a treat. The entire line has been updated in recent years, but the perennial favorites remain, such as the feminine Alexandra fragrance and the incomparable Countess Isserlyn foundations. These long-lasting, flawless foundations are particularly favored by the Hollywood movie community. Look for ads featuring supermodel Patti Hansen, with the tagline: "For Women. Not For Girls."

The Alexandra scent is also available in luxurious body powder and body lotion, and is surprisingly well-priced.

Introduced   1979
Price   Mid-range

ALFRED SUNG
E.N.C.O.R.E.

Scent Type
    Floral - Oriental
Composition
    Top Notes: *Tangerine, ylang-ylang, Grasse neroli*
    Heart Notes: *Jasmine absolute, tuberose absolute, mousse de Chine, Oriental rose oil*
    Base Notes: *Indian sandalwood oil, musk accord, patchouli, vanilla, incense*

E.N.C.O.R.E. is an elegant floral bouquet with exotic base notes that creator and fashion designer Alfred Sung describes in these words: "...feminine and romantic yet vibrant and dynamic." Sung's fragrances are manufactured and distributed worldwide through the dynamic reach of Riviera Concepts, an international team of fragrance pros.

The subtle "floriental" scent of E.N.C.O.R.E. begins with a light touch of tangerine and florals, followed by rich, beautiful floral essences of rose, jasmine and tuberose. Long-lasting Oriental notes of sandalwood, vanilla and musk complete the understated arrangement. A lovely, ultra-feminine fragrance, from day to evening.

The curved flacon is a graceful design by Pierre Dinand, featuring frosted-tipped shoulders and a sculpted stopper. Packaging, in marbleized dove grey with red accents, epitomizes the refinement and elegance for which Alfred Sung is known. The Exquisite Bath and Body Collection is available to layer and lengthen the fragrance experience. Pure indulgence.

Introduced   1990
Price   High range

ALFRED SUNG SPA

Scent Type
    Green
Composition
    Top Notes: *Orange Guinea, bergamot, lemon, mandarin, galbanum, ylang-ylang*
    Heart Notes: *Calone, tropical jasmine, muguet, hyacinth, orange blossom, rose, geranium*
    Base Notes: *Sandalwood, musk*

Alfred Sung Spa is a light, fresh fragrance one can experience in a line of spa ritual products, including scented foam bath, shampoo, lotions, masks, body spray, and sun protectors. The entire collection is designed to soothe, renew and refresh from head to toe.

Sung Spa thrills with an effervescent citrus top note for a sparkling clean beginning, followed by florals and greens, including muguet, or lily of the valley. More casual than other Sung fragrances, Sung Spa is a fresh, uplifting scent for active days and warm summer evenings; a beautiful morning fragrance.

In keeping with the healthy theme, Sung Spa is housed in clean white, recyclable bottles and is color coded to reflect the mood of each product. Printed materials are on recycled paper printed with vegetable ink. Products are all-natural and biodegradable, and are not tested on animals.

Sung says: "True serenity comes to those who seek it....Fundamentals for your healthy mind and body." Makes us want to slip into the Spa foam bath right now...go ahead...and take a good book...preferably this one....

Introduced	*1992*
Price	*Mid-range*

ALIAGE

Scent Type
  Chypre - Green
Composition
  Top Notes: Greens, peach, citrus oils
  Heart Notes: Jasmine, rosewood, pine, thyme
  Base Notes: Oakmoss, musk, vetiver, myrrh

Aliage is a green chypre blend of more than 300 ingredients from Estée Lauder. Reportedly the aroma of fresh palm leaves served as inspiration for the sporty scent, which Lauder created for casual active wear. It is said she was searching for a light fragrance suitable for a midday tennis game.

The remarkable story of Estée Lauder began with a skin treatment creme formula that spawned the signature line of color cosmetics, skin care and fragrance, as well as the Prescriptives, Clinique, Aramis and Lauder for Men lines. Other Lauder activities include the Estée and Joseph H. Lauder Foundation, along with the endowment of the Lauder Institute for International Studies at the Wharton School of Business, University of Pennsylvania. Today the Lauder empire is still a family business with son Leonard and his wife Evelyn at the helm, assisted by other talented family members. The company serves as a shining example of what one woman can accomplish.

Introduced	*1972*
Price	*Mid-range*

AMARIGE

Scent Type
Floral - Fruity
Composition
Top Notes: Mandarin, neroli,
violet leaves, rosewood
Heart Notes: Gardenia, red fruits,
ylang-ylang, acacia farnesiana, mimosa
Base Notes: Musk, vanilla, tonka bean,
woods, ambergris

Amarige is the latest offering from
French couturier Hubert de Givenchy.
According to him, it is designed to conjure up
images of "...mirages and magic...amorous,
marvelous encounters and marriage...a tribute
to youthful exuberance."

Amarige is a romantic floral creation,
youthful and fresh, lightened by sparkling notes
of mandarin and neroli, followed by rich white
flowers embedded in a sensual musk, wood and
vanilla base. A delicately feminine fragrance.

The bottle was reportedly inspired by a
soft yellow organza blouse from the Givenchy
couture collection. The frosted glass flacon is
naturally curved and presented in packaging
bearing the familiar Givenchy 4-G imprint.

For a treat, try the Amarige bath and
body line, luxurious products chock-full of
sweet almond oil, allantoin, collagen, vitamin
E, coconut oil, jojoba oil and more.

Introduced   *1992*
Price   *High range*

AMAZONE

Scent Type
Floral - Fruity
Composition
Top Notes: Lemon, orange, bergamot,
peach, strawberry, grapefruit, tangerine,
galbanum
Heart Notes: Daffodil, hyacinth,
narcissus, black currant bud, iris, jasmine,
raspberry, lily of the valley
Base Notes: Sandalwood, vetiver,
cedarwood, neroli, ylang-ylang, oakmoss

Amazone is from Hermès, the Parisian
maker of fine leathers, silks, porcelains, fashions
and more since 1837. Amazone is a modern
floral bouquet with lively top notes of fruity
citrus, most notably orange, lemon, raspberry
and black currant bud. The delicate floral heart
is formed with hyacinth, jasmine and narcissus
amid a proliferation of other floral essences.
Ideal for liberal daytime use.

Hermès describes Amazone as "tender and
impetuous," a playful fragrance, full of romance
and charm. The second women's fragrance
developed by Hermès, Amazone is packaged in
a vivid orange-red box, nestled in a print silk
paper. Also available in body and bath products.

Introduced   *1974*
Price   *Top range*

AMOUR AMOUR

Scent Type
   Floral - Fresh
Composition
   Top Notes: *Bergamot, strawberry,*
   lemon, neroli
   Heart Notes: *Jasmine, narcissus, rose,*
   ylang-ylang, carnation, oregano, lily
   Base Notes: *Vetiver, honey, musk,*
   civet, heliotrope

The first perfume from French couturier
Jean Patou, Amour Amour was an instant
success in chic 1925 Paris circles. The name
refers to the first moment of love, the instant
when the heartbeat quickens. Amour Amour
was the first of the love trilogy scents com-
memorating the three great stages of love, a trio
of Patou fragrances that includes Que sais-je?,
meaning "What do I know?" and representing
the instant of hesitation, and Adieu Sagesse, or
"Farewell wisdom," the time of surrender. (For
more information on Que sais-je? and Adieu
Sagesse, see the Ma Collection Profile.) A rich
fragrance of comfort and luxury, its seductive
multi-floral notes are lightened with a tangy top
note of bergamot.

The haute couture House of Jean Patou
opened in 1919, catering to the changing trends
of an increasingly mobile and active wealthy
class. Patou was on the crest of the 1920s
introduction of modern sportswear, with his
slimming bathing suits and sun products for the
newly emerging sun worshippers—tremendous
hits across the Mediterranean sands. Always

at the forefront of fashion, he was the first to
stamp his monogram on his designs, sparking
a designer label trend that has spanned decades.
In 1925, Patou swept to American shores and
enjoyed similar success as the first French
couturier to employ American models and
design specifically for the American woman.

For more insight into the vintage fragrances
of the dapper Jean Patou, see the Ma Collection
Profile in this book. It outlines twelve of
Patou's most popular fragrances, re-created and
packaged as a set.

Introduced   1925
Price   Mid-range

ANAÏS ANAÏS

Scent Type
   Floral - Fresh
Composition
   Top Notes: *White Madonna lily, black*
   currant bud, hyacinth, lily of the valley, citrus
   Heart Notes: *Moroccan jasmine, Grasse rose,*
   Florentine iris, Madagascar ylang-ylang and
   orange blossom, Bourbon vetiver,
   California cedarwood, Singapore patchouli,
   Yugoslavian oakmoss
   Base Notes: *Russian leather, musk*

Anaïs Anaïs is a nostalgic floral blend,
delicate, soft and subtle. French couturier Jean
Bousquet, founder of Cacharel describes his
fragrance in these words: "Anaïs Anaïs is a

65

perfume whose essence is romanticism with the scent of lilies. It has been housed in opaque jars reminiscent of the ancient world." The white jars bear a peach floral motif, created by bottle designer Annegret Beier. Anaïs Anaïs is an ideal scent for the young and the young at heart, those who are gentle and feminine in nature.

The innocence of the scent is created by the dominant note of white lilies, called Madonna lilies, cultivated in the south of France, Bulgaria and the Middle East. Greeks and Romans considered this lily a symbol of purity. Each lily produces a few drops of the precious essence; in fact, one ton of petals produces only one pound of lily oil.

The scent is available in a wide range of fragrance, bath and body products. A new item, Voile de Parfum, is an alcohol-free moisturizing perfume, subtle as the eau de toilette, but richer and longer lasting. The perfume oils are diluted in liposomes, a patented hydrating and moisturizing formula, rather than alcohol.

Bousquet clearly takes pleasure in selecting interesting names. He borrowed the name of his company, Cacharel, from the wild ducks native to Provence. And Anaïs Anaïs? The fragrance is named after the Persian Goddess of Love.

Introduced	*1978*
Price	*Mid-range*

ANDIAMO

Scent Type
Floral - Green

Composition
Top Notes: Rose, ylang-ylang, jasmine, citrus, greens
Heart Notes: Clove, cinnamon
Base Notes: Oakmoss, greens, patchouli, amber

Andiamo is a brisk, spirited fragrance from Princess Marcella Borghese. The fragrance is a smooth blend of citrus, greens, florals, spices and woods. The result is a fresh green floral, ideal for sports and warm summer evenings. Quite fitting, for in Italian, Andiamo means "on the move."

Introduced	*1970*
Price	*Mid-range*

ANGEL

Scent Type
Oriental
Composition
Top Notes: Fruits, dewberry, helonial, honey
Heart Notes: Chocolate, caramel, coumarin
Base Notes: Vanilla, patchouli

Famous Patrons
Diana Ross

Futuristic fashion designer Thierry Mugler is wishing upon a star with his first fragrance, Angel. The blue-colored essence is an Oriental composition, with fragrance notes that sound more like dessert ingredients: chocolate, caramel, honey and vanilla. Mugler says the scent is meant to stir "innocent childhood memories." Sensual wooded notes provide the adult theme.

Mugler explains his ambition: "I wanted a mouthwatering fragrance that also had strength and punch, just like my designs—my suits can be cut sharp and tight, yet molded to the feminine curve. It's called Angel because angels bring about dreams and the imaginary; they are a mystery; powerful, yet soft."

Angel comes in heavenly packaging. Mugler's personal symbol is the star, evidenced by his star-shaped ring and tattoo. The elongated five-pointed star flacon is produced by glassmaker Brosse in heavy glass of brilliant blue, and is refillable, as well as recyclable.

Catch a falling star with Angel, Mugler's rising star.

Introduced   1993
Price   High range

ANIMALE

Scent Type
    Chypre - Floral
Composition
    Top Notes: *Neroli, bergamot, hyacinth, coriander, greens*
    Heart Notes: *Jasmine, rose, pimento berry, ylang-ylang*
    Base Notes: *Patchouli, vetiver, musk, labdanum, oakmoss*

Animale is a chypre floral bouquet of rare essential oils from Suzanne de Lyon. The brilliant scent is matched only by the vivid packaging in fuchsia, amber, emerald and teal.

The captivating scent of Animale is also available in a luxurious bath and body collection: dusting powder, body lotion, foaming gel and body creme.

Introduced   1987
Price   High range

ANNE KLEIN

Scent Type
    Floral
Composition
    Top Notes: *Greens, galbanum, hyacinth, neroli, cassie, bergamot, aldehydes*
    Heart Notes: *Bulgarian rose, mandarin, lily of the valley, jasmine, orchid, rose*
    Base Notes: *Sandalwood, vetiver, vanilla, amber, benzoin, musk, civet*

The original signature fragrance from contemporary New York fashion designer Anne Klein is a modern floral blend, light and easy to wear. Green and aldehydic top notes impart a fresh lift, while the final impression is of powdery florals and woods.

Introduced   1984
Price   High range

ANNE KLEIN II

Scent Type
   Oriental - Ambery
Composition
   Top Notes: *Peach, rosewood, greens, lemon*
   Heart Notes: *Lily, jasmine, rose,*
   orange blossom, ylang-ylang, orris, carnation
   Base Notes: *Vanilla, amber, sandalwood,*
   musk, patchouli, civet, benzoin

The sequel from Anne Klein is an exotic Oriental melange of flowers, spices and sweet amber. The scent is vivid, spicy, sophisticated and long-lasting. A lovely complement to the original fragrance, it is also available in soothing body and bath products.

Introduced	*1986*
Price	*High range*

ANTILOPE

Scent Type
   Floral - Aldehyde
Composition
   Top Notes: *Grasse neroli, bergamot,*
   chamomile, sage, aldehydes
   Heart Notes: *Lily of the valley, jasmine*
   Base Notes: *Patchouli, iris, ambergris, vetiver*

Antilope is a classic French floral fragrance dating from the Roaring Twenties, created by the couture House of Weil.

The floral melange is introduced by crisp citrus notes of bergamot and neroli, enhanced with a brilliant touch of aldehydes poised against a sensual backdrop of warm chypre woods, patchouli and vetiver, with a sprinkling of spicy iris. Chamomile contributes a soothing note.

The resulting Antilope fragrance is a sophisticated, enduring floral, with a lingering aura of deep forest woods.

Introduced	*1928*
Price	*Mid-range*

ANTONIA'S FLOWERS

Scent Type
   Floral
Composition
   Notes: *Freesia, jasmine, lily of the valley,*
   magnolia, fruits

A delightful bouquet of flowers is gathered in Antonia's Flowers. The delicate composition is based on the fresh scent of freesia and enhanced by a selection of spring flowers and fruits. A light fragrance, Antonia's Flowers is suitable for casual daytime and warm weather wear, afternoon tea, or a late evening walk on the beach.

"I imagined a perfume that would evoke the sensation of entering my flower shop," says creator Antonia Bellanca. She selected the dominant note of freesia for its clean, innocent aroma. She first discovered and fell in love with freesia as an art student in France. And now, she has put the flowers in a bottle.

Packaged in rectangular glass flacons, Antonia's Flowers is decorated with pastel watercolor sketches of wildflowers. The scent is also available in body lotion, bath gel and twice-milled soaps.

Introduced   1982
Price   Mid-range

APRÈS L'ONDÉE

Scent Type
   Floral - Ambery
Composition
   Top Notes: *Violet, bergamot, cassie, neroli*
   Heart Notes: *Carnation, ylang-ylang, iris, rose, jasmine, mimosa, vetiver, sandalwood*
   Base Notes: *Vanilla, musk, amber, heliotrope*

A graceful creation by Jacques Guerlain, Après L'Ondée is described by the company as "an inspired portrait of the most delicate imaginary flower." Elusively charming, fresh and sparkling, it is a refined floral bouquet with a sweet amber base, suitable for most any occasion. Après L'Ondée is one of more than 300 scents developed by the renowned House of Guerlain.

The House of Guerlain is the world's oldest family-owned fragrance and cosmetic company. Spanning five generations, it was founded in 1828 by doctor and chemist Pierre-François-Pascal Guerlain. The shop was first located on the rue de Rivoli in Paris, then moved to No. 15 rue de la Paix, where young Guerlain

created his hallmark—personalized fragrances in sync with the wearer's personality, fragrances that often lived for only one evening or event. Writer Honoré de Balzac commissioned a custom-blended scent during the writing of *César Birotteau*, and Empress Eugénie named Guerlain perfumer to the Napoléonic court, for which many Empire fragrances were created. In fact, Guerlain was appointed perfumer to most of the royal courts of Europe, including those of the Empress of Austria and the Queens of England, Spain and Romania.

Introduced   1906
Price   High range

AROMATICS ELIXIR

Scent Type
   Chypre - Floral
Composition
   Top Notes: *Chamomile, orange blossom, bergamot, coriander, rosewood, aldehydes, greens, palmarosa*
   Heart Notes: *Jasmine, rose, ylang-ylang, tuberose, orris, carnation*
   Base Notes: *Sandalwood, oakmoss, vetiver, patchouli, musk, cistus, civet*

Aromatics Elixir is designed to soothe and subtly stimulate, with notes of gentle chamomile and sweet sandalwood set against a classic blend of French florals and aromatic woods. The dominant chypre theme is a natural accord enhanced by juicy citrus and lawn greens.

Introduced   1971
Price   Mid-range

ARPÈGE

Scent Type
Floral - Aldehyde
Composition
Top Notes: *Bergamot, neroli, aldehydes, peach*
Heart Notes: *Rose, jasmine, ylang-ylang,
lily of the valley*
Base Notes: *Sandalwood, vetiver, patchouli,
vanilla, musk*

Famous Patrons
Jacqueline Bisset
Princess Diana of Wales

Arpège is a restoration and reformulation
of the original 1927 scent from French couturier
Jeanne Lanvin and perfumer Andre Fraysse.
The reborn scent was introduced in France and
Belgium in 1993 and scheduled for launch in
North America in 1994 or 1995.

More than sixty natural essences are housed
in the classic ball-shaped flacon, or *boule noire*.
A black opaque glass bottle houses the perfume,
while the eau de parfum resides in a clear glass
bottle. A gold-colored image of Jeanne Lanvin
and her daughter Marie-Blanche dressing for a
ball is stamped on the glass, just as it was on the
original bottles. The fragrance was christened
Arpège for its similarity to the musical arpeggio
—a tumble of notes in quick succession. The
result is an elegant floral composition with a
sensual wooded finish.

The Parisian House of Lanvin was founded
by Jeanne Lanvin. She created the popular
mother-daughter design concept, in addition
to designing evening gowns, bridal wear and
menswear. After Lanvin's death in 1946,
daughter Marie-Blanche, also known as the
Comtesse de Polignac, continued the business
with Bernard Lanvin.

The relaunch of Arpège coincided with the
remodeling of Lanvin's boutiques on the rue du
Faubourg Saint Honoré. How we love to see
the classics revived. Welcome back, Arpège.

Introduced   1927
Relaunched   1993
Price   Mid-range

ASJA

Scent Type
Floral - Oriental
Composition
Top Notes: *Fruits, citrus*
Heart Notes: *Bulgarian rose,
Egyptian jasmine, ylang-ylang, cinnamon,
nutmeg, mimosa*
Base Notes: *Sandalwood, musk,
vanilla, amber*

Asja is a fragrant creation from the House
of Fendi, the Roman empire ruled by five Fendi
sisters. Carla Fendi states, "The dream of any
design house is to have its own proper fragrance,
because when a woman gets dressed, the final
touch is her fragrance."

A dramatic, sensual fragrance, Asja represents the meeting of East and West. The Fendi family drew upon its own Turkish heritage in developing the scent, a rich floral Oriental that unfolds beneath fresh fruity top notes.

The Eastern influence extends to the distinctive Fendi gold-colored and black striped packaging, likened to a molded Chinese lacquer box. The exotic juice is captured in brilliant red bottles.

In Asja, as in the Orient, Fendi says, "fantasy rules and illusion seduces."

Introduced	*1993 (1992 Italy)*
Price	*Top range*

AZURÉE

Scent Type
   Chypre - Floral Animalic
Composition
   Top Notes: *Bergamot, aldehydes, gardenia, artemisia*
   Heart Notes: *Jasmine, geranium, ylang-ylang, orris, cyclamen*
   Base Notes: *Leather, oakmoss, patchouli, musk, amber*

Azurée is a chypre floral melody from Estée Lauder, said to have been inspired by the tangy Mediterranean bergamot fruit, an inedible fruit prized for perfumery.

The fragrance features herbal and aldehydic top notes, dry floral heart notes and woody base notes redolent of warm leather and moss. Azurée is a versatile everyday scent.

Introduced	*1969*
Price	*Mid-range*

AZZARO

Scent Type
   Chypre - Fruity
Composition
   Top Notes: *Fruits, gardenias, aldehydes*
   Heart Notes: *Jasmine, rose, ylang-ylang, orris*
   Base Notes: *Moss, styrax, amber, vetiver, patchouli*

From couturier Loris Azzaro comes his original signature fragrance, presented in a circular perfume flacon rimmed in jet black.

Born in Tunisia, Azzaro became known in Paris for his exclusive collections of sensual evening wear. His splendid gowns have graced the figures of actresses Sophia Loren and Marisa Berenson.

The fragrance evolves from an initial blend of fruits and aldehydes to a floral heart that rests on a base accord of mossy balsamics. The result is like a springtime frolic through moist grassy fields of sun-ripened fruit trees.

Introduced	*1984*
Price	*Mid-range*

AZZARO 9

Scent Type
Floral

Composition
Top Notes: *Pineapple, aldehydes, mandarin, bergamot*
Heart Notes: *Jasmine, foxglove, tulip, wisteria, clematis, lily, mimosa, rose, orange blossom*
Base Notes: *Sandalwood, cedarwood, musk, moss, vanilla*

Azzaro 9 is a feminine floral bouquet with a dominant accord of nine yellow and white flowers, created by Loris Azzaro. Fruity green top notes give way to a floral heart that dries down to a powdery wooded finish.

In England, the 1993 Chelsea Flower Show paid tribute to Azzaro. For the show, Lord Kenilworth of the *Sunday Times* designed a landscape using the nine main flowers of the Azzaro 9 fragrance. Must have been lovely!

Azzaro 9 is presented in a graceful Pierre Dinand-designed bottle and packaging of dazzling yellow and white, just like the bouquet of flowers it contains. The perfect fragrance to accent an exotic Azzaro-designed evening gown.

Introduced	*1986*
Price	*Mid-range*

BAL à VERSAILLES

Scent Type
Oriental - Ambery Spicy

Composition
Top Notes: *Grasse jasmine, Bulgarian rose, Anatolian rose, May rose, Farnesian cassie*
Heart Notes: *Sandalwood, patchouli, vetiver*
Base Notes: *Musk, ambergris, gums, resins, civet*

Famous Patrons
Elizabeth Taylor

Bal à Versailles is a classic French fragrance from the legendary Parisian perfumer Jean Desprez. More than 350 rare essences were used to create the long-lasting, dramatic fragrance. A rich and feminine Oriental blend, it features florals, ambers, spices and sweet balsamic base notes. Bal à Versailles is ideal for sophisticated day wear and elegant evenings.

In the thirties, Jean Desprez established his perfumery on the prestigious rue de la Paix in Paris, serving an exclusive clientele. Besides his popular Bal à Versailles, he also created Grand Dame, Étourdissant and Vôtre Main in 1939, Jardanel in 1972, and Révolution à Versailles. Upon his death in 1973, he was succeeded by his son Denis Desprez and daughter Marie Celine Garnier.

Bal à Versailles is presented in an array of classic fragrance flacons. Our favorite is a round decanter with a label featuring a romantic party scene; no doubt it is from the most famous dance or "ball" of Versailles—the Bal à Versailles. This scene is a miniature reproduction of a

Fragonard painting that is part of the Sevres Museum collection. The scene also appeared on a porcelain dish by Madame Ducluzeau known as *La Coupe des Sens*, or "cup of the senses," featuring miniatures representing the five senses. When Desprez was searching for inspiration, he spied the cup and was intrigued by the Fragonard scene, which was included to represent the sense of smell. *Quel appropos!*

Introduced	*1962*
Price	*Mid-range*

BALAHÉ

Scent Type
> *Floral - Ambery*

Composition
> **Top Notes:** *Bergamot, mandarin, clary sage, coriander, pineapple, plum*
> **Heart Notes:** *Rose, jasmine, ylang-ylang, tuberose, orange blossom, orchid*
> **Base Notes:** *Vanilla, vetiver, sandalwood, musk, civet*

From Léonard Parfums Paris comes Balahé, a striking floral with ambery Oriental base notes in an equally striking flacon—sculpted black clasped with a red rope—a Serge Mansau design. Balahé is a dramatic statement, not for the timid.

Designer Philippe Léonard founded Léonard Parfums in 1969, building on the success of his *prêt-à-porter* collection. Balahé is his fourth women's fragrance, after Fashion, Eau Fraîche and Tamango.

Introduced	*1987*
Price	*Mid-range*

BANDIT

Scent Type
> *Chypre - Floral Animalic*

Composition
> **Top Notes:** *Artemisia, bergamot, gardenia, aldehydes*
> **Heart Notes:** *Jasmine, orris, rose, carnation*
> **Base Notes:** *Moss, castoreum, patchouli, amber, vetiver, civet, myrrh*

Bandit is a classic fragrance developed during World War II by couturier Robert Piguet. It is a delightful blend of dry herbs and florals with a long-lasting base of aromatic woods, mosses and warm leather.

Swiss-born Piguet apprenticed under couturier Paul Poiret in glamorous 1920 Paris. By 1928 he had his own salon, specializing in couture creations for petite, youthful women. He trained the next generation of designers at his salon: Pierre Balmain, Hubert de Givenchy, Castillo, James Galanos. Christian Dior once said that he learned from Piguet "the virtues of simplicity...how to suppress."

How to catch a Bandit?...Look for it dressed in pared-down Piguet black, naturally.

Introduced	*1944*
Price	*Mid-range*

BASIC BLACK

Scent Type
  Floral - Fruity
Composition
  Top Notes: Bergamot, mandarin,
  ylang-ylang, cardamom
  Heart Notes: Rose, violet, coriander
  Base Notes: Patchouli, oakmoss, sandalwood

Basic Black is one of a trio of fragrances (along with Nude and Hot) that Bill Blass introduced in 1990. Perhaps Basic Black was named in honor of the little black dress, a perennial basic in any well-dressed woman's wardrobe.

Basic Black begins with fruity top notes of crisp bergamot and smooth mandarin. A floral bouquet is enhanced by soft wooded base notes. The result is a subtle daytime fragrance, as basic as the little black dress.

Introduced   1990
Price   High range

BEAUTIFUL

Scent Type
  Floral

Composition
  Top Notes: Bergamot, galbanum, lemon,
  cassie, fruits
  Heart Notes: Rose, ylang-ylang, lilac, violet,
  lily of the valley, carnation, sage, geranium,
  rose violet, narcissus, orange blossom, mimosa,
  marigold, freesia, chamomile, tuberose,
  jasmine, neroli, jonquil, magnolia
  Base Notes: Sandalwood, vetiver, musk,
  vanilla, cedarwood

Beautiful is a romantic scent from Estée Lauder, bursting with a cornucopia of fruit and wildflower essences. The fragrance was designed to embody femininity, softness and romance, like a goddess floating through a cloud of white. Lauder reportedly received her inspiration for the fragrance from the gardens of Giverny, the same gardens that inspired Monet.

The bottle, from I. Levy-Alain Carré, is a study in classic simplicity, a vessel of clear glass inscribed with the name Beautiful. It rests easily in the hand and travels well. Like wildflowers, Beautiful blossoms in the springtime sun.

Introduced   1985
Price   Mid-range

BELLODGIA

Scent Type
  Floral
Composition
  Top and Heart Notes: Rose, jasmine,
  lily of the valley
  Base Notes: Spicy carnation

Bellodgia is a classic 1920s fragrance from the notable French fragrance house Parfums Caron. The fragrance takes its name from a romantic island on Lake Como in Northern Italy. The feminine floral bouquet is distinguished by a rich accord of rose and jasmine accenting the dominant theme of spicy carnation. A chic, sophisticated perfume.

Parfums Caron was established in Paris in 1904 to introduce fragrances created by master perfumer Ernest Daltroff. Today, Parfums Caron presents its timeless fragrances on the fashionable avenue Montaigne in Paris. The store is a sight to behold—each exquisite Caron fragrance floats in Louis XV-style Baccarat crystal flacons, from which you can draw the amount of fragrance you desire. For a special treat, a limited edition Baccarat flacon filled with three ounces of Bellodgia can be yours for a mere $1,700. Elsewhere, look for Bellodgia prepackaged in perfume and eau de toilette fragrance strengths.

Introduced	*1927*
Price	*High range*

BIJAN

Scent Type
  Floral - Oriental
Composition
  Top Notes: *Ylang-ylang, narcissus, orange blossom*
  Heart Notes: *Persian jasmine, Bulgarian rose, lily of the valley*
  Base Notes: *Moroccan oakmoss, sandalwood, patchouli*

Famous Patrons
  Oprah Winfrey
  Queen Elizabeth II

A floral Oriental with soft fruity top notes, Bijan is the original signature fragrance from Bijan, prominent Beverly Hills menswear designer. He is featured in his own flamboyant, award-winning ads with Niki, his exclusive raven-haired spokesmodel and muse.

Two-and-a-half years in the making, the fragrance is composed of rich seductive florals poised against exotic woods, creating a refined, feminine statement.

From kings to presidents to the simply wealthy, Bijan's clients seek out his inimitable style at his "by appointment only" Rodeo Drive showroom and boutique. Of course, there is an adjacent Bijan fragrance boutique for quick trips...or visit the New York and London boutiques. The fragrance can also be found at the finest department stores and perfumeries.

The scent is packaged in a round bottle with a hole in the center, designed by Bijan and made originally by Pouchet of France. The design garnered a 1993 Clear Choice Award from the Glass Packaging Institute. Bijan donated his $1,000 cash award to UNICEF, an honor accepted by UNICEF spokeswoman and *Hill Street Blues* actress Barbara Bochco.

Introduced	*1987*
Price	*Top range*

BILL BLASS

Scent Type
  Floral
Composition
  Top Notes: *Galbanum, hyacinth, pineapple, greens, bergamot, geranium*
  Heart Notes: *Iris, tuberose, carnation, ylang-ylang, orris*
  Base Notes: *Amber, sandalwood, benzoin, cedarwood, oakmoss*

From American designer Bill Blass comes a classic floral bouquet. Like his clothing designs, the fragrance is subtle, elegant...uniquely Blass. A feminine scent, featuring sweet fruits, florals, amber and wood notes. An excellent choice for daytime or light evening wear.

Introduced   1978
Price   High range

BLUE GRASS

Scent Type
  Floral - Ambery
Composition
  Top Notes: *Aldehydes, lavender, orange, neroli, bergamot*
  Heart Notes: *Jasmine, tuberose, narcissus, rose, carnation*
  Base Notes: *Sandalwood, musk, tonka bean, benzoin*

Famous Patrons
  Queen Elizabeth II

Six decades ago, Elizabeth Arden introduced her Blue Grass. Still as lovely today, Blue Grass is an enduring, easy-to-wear classic, ideal for casual, professional or daytime wear. Surprisingly well-priced, too.

Elizabeth Arden was an early entrepreneur in the American cosmetics industry. Born Florence Graham in Ontario, Canada, she derived her professional name from a favorite book: *Elizabeth and Her German Garden.* As a nurse, she developed a skin care regime that became popular in her beauty salons, the first of which opened its red door in New York in 1910. Her love of nature and flowers moved her to create fragrance and inspired the name for Blue Grass, after the shimmering view of verdant fields visible from the windows of her Virginia home.

Introduced   1934
Price   Mid-range

BOIS DES ÎLES

Scent Type
  Floral - Aldehyde
Composition
  Top Notes: *Bergamot, petitgrain, coriander, aldehydes*
  Heart Notes: *Jasmine, rose, ylang-ylang, iris*
  Base Notes: *Vetiver, amber, sandalwood, tonka bean*

In the 1920s, French couturier Gabrielle "Coco" Chanel collaborated with the great perfumer Ernest Beaux to create the Chanel scents that have become legend: No. 5, No. 19 and No. 22. Now, Chanel reintroduces a trio of exhilarating fragrances from the twenties: Bois des Îles, Cuir de Russie and Gardenia.

The woody floral blend of Bois des Îles begins with top notes of fresh citrus, spice and sparkling aldehydes entwined with rich florals and sweet lasting woods. A subtly sensual fragrance, understated and understood.

Bois des Îles, or "wood of the isles," is a welcome return to an era of grace and elegance. Look for it exclusively in Chanel Boutiques.

Introduced	*1926*
Reintroduced	*1993*
Price	*Mid-range*

BOUCHERON

Scent Type
  Floral Semi-Oriental
Composition
  Top Notes: *Sicilian tangerine, Calabrian bitter orange, apricot, Persian galbanum, African tagetes, Spanish basilica*
  Heart Notes: *Moroccan orange blossom, Grasse tuberose, Madagascar ylang-ylang, Moroccan jasmine, Auvergne narcissus, British broom*
  Base Notes: *Mysore sandalwood, amber, Indian Ocean vanilla, South American tonka bean*

Boucheron is the signature fragrance from the renowned French jeweler Frederic Boucheron. The delicate, feminine scent is introduced by lively green and fruity top notes, then develops into an intense heart of sensual florals. Underscoring the arrangement are warm, woody background notes, sensual and long-lasting.

The first Boucheron jewelry store was established more than a century ago by Frederic Boucheron in the exclusive Palais Royal section of Paris. The store can now be found in the famous Place Vendôme of Paris, as well as in Geneva, London, Tokyo, Gstaad and North American cities. In 1988, descendant Alain Boucheron moved into the universe of fragrance to create jewelry for the senses. He combined the craftsmanship of the jeweler with the art of the perfumer to produce the fragrance, a scent designed to exude elegance, mystery and allure, as a reflection of legendary Boucheron jewels.

The fragrance swirls in an oval ring-shaped bottle. The flacons are made in France, carved from rock crystal and ringed with golden orbs, called gadroons. The fragrant ornament is crowned in deep blue Burmese sapphire. The lovely package echoes Boucheron jewelry designs of soft sculpted curves. In 1989, the fragrance industry honored Boucheron with two prestigious FiFi Awards, one for best packaging and one for best fragrance in its distribution category.

Boucheron...a beautiful, artistic marriage of French perfume and French jewelry.

Introduced	*1988*
Price	*Top range*

BULGARI EAU PARFUMÉE

Scent Type
 Floral
Composition
 Top Notes: *Italian bergamot, Spanish orange blossom, Ceylonese cardamom, Jamaican pepper, Russian coriander*
 Heart Notes: *Bulgarian Rose, Egyptian jasmine*
 Base Notes: *Green tea, woods*

In 1993, world-renowned jeweler Bulgari introduced its first fragrance. The initial impression is fresh and fruity with zesty bergamot, quickly followed by soft notes of spicy coriander and pepper. After a few minutes, the fragrance develops into a warm floral heart of rose and jasmine. The lingering aroma is a soothing blend of florals with exotic woods and spices, plus an unusual component, the essence of green tea.

The history behind the fragrance revolves around Ming-Le, the philosophy of the Chinese tea ceremony. In Chinese, Ming-Le means "the joy of tea" and, according to Bulgari, denotes "honoring meditation, the time for a break" and "the respect of one's own rhythm," representing "a philosophy of life where understatement and discretion play a leading role." It is based on "the art of living, and the act of giving oneself pleasure, beauty and joy." Tea symbolizes harmony and purity and is the important base note of the Bulgari fragrance.

The scent is presented in a curved rectangular flacon of pale green frosted glass, in recycled and biodegradable packaging.

The fragrance was initially available only at Bulgari stores. The flagship store is in Rome, on the prestigious via Condotti. Other locations include New York, Paris, Geneva, Monte Carlo, Beverly Hills and Las Vegas at The Caesars Forum. Today the descendants of founder Sotirio Bulgari, an 1879 Greek immigrant to Italy, still manage the artisans who blend the elegant styles of the Mediterranean and Italian Renaissance into fine Bulgari jewelry, noted for its quality, volume, purity and smoothness.

Introduced 1993
Price *High range*

BYBLOS

Scent Type
 Floral - Fruity
Composition
 Top Notes: *Mandarin, grapefruit, cassie, marigold, bergamot, peach*
 Heart Notes: *Honeysuckle, gardenia, mimosa, ylang-ylang, lily of the valley, orchid, rose, heliotrope, violet, orris*
 Base Notes: *Musk, vetiver, pepper, raspberry*

Imported from Milan, Byblos is a floral bouquet inspired by the magic of the Mediterranean and its ancient cultures. The memorable scent combines tangy fruits, fragrant florals, fresh greens and light lingering woods.

Byblos is housed in a bottle of brilliant Mediterranean blue, crowned with a carved apricot blossom. Look for the related line of Byblos fashions.

Introduced   1992
Price   Mid-range

BYZANCE

Scent Type
> Floral Semi-Oriental

Composition
> **Top Notes:** Citrus, cardamom, spices, greens, mandarin, aldehydes, basil
> **Heart Notes:** Jasmine, tuberose, Turkish rose, lily of the valley, ylang-ylang
> **Base Notes:** Sandalwood, vanilla, musk, heliotrope, amber

Byzance is a 1980s creation from Parfums Rochas. Inspired by the meeting between Eastern and Western cultures, the semi-Oriental blend contains rare essences from all over the globe.

The initial impression of Byzance is one of soft fruits and fresh aldehydes. Ephemeral and airy, it sets the stage for the delicate floral bouquet. The drydown notes are subtly rendered as refined sandalwood is blended with the tenacity of vanilla and musk. The result is an understated composition with a magnificent trail, that certain something that makes people turn and wonder, "What was she wearing?" A tasteful fragrance, suitable for most any occasion, day to evening.

The round flacon, designed by In-House, draws heavily from Baroque art. The crystal decanter is the deepest Mediterranean blue, gilded with a seal that contains the name Byzance thrice sculpted in relief. A fuchsia ribbon encircles the slender neck. One of the most beautiful bottles we've seen, it echoes the opulence, femininity and sensuality of the fragrance itself.

Introduced   1986
Price   High range

C'EST LA VIE!

Scent Type
> Floral - Ambery

Composition
> **Top Notes:** Bergamot, orange blossom, pineapple, peach, aldehydes
> **Heart Notes:** Ylang-ylang, carnation, jasmine, rose, tuberose, heliotrope, orris
> **Base Notes:** Amber, vanilla, cedarwood, sandalwood, musk

Famous Patrons
> Ivana Trump

C'est la vie! is a sensual fragrance from the ultra-creative Parisian couturier Christian Lacroix. The bright, exhilarating floral bouquet is warmed by long-lasting amber notes.

C'est la vie! is presented in a coral branch-style flacon by designer Maurice Roger and tucked inside a jewel-tone satin pouch. A sophisticated salute to the good life.

Introduced   1986
Price   High range

CABOCHARD

Scent Type
Chypre - Floral Animalic

Composition
Top Notes: Citrus, aldehydes, fruits, spices
Heart Notes: Jasmine, rose, ylang-ylang, orris, geranium
Base Notes: Leather, tobacco, amber, patchouli, musk, moss, vetiver, castoreum

Originally introduced in 1959, the classic Cabochard from the Parisian House of Grès is a delightful chypre blend of citrus, mosses and dry florals.

Mme Grès was born Alix Barton and became known for her fluid designs that draped the body. Twice she had to close her salon doors during World War II, but in 1946 she reestablished the House of Grès, along with the fashions and the fragrances that remain with us today.

Legend has it that Mme Grès had taken a trip through the Spice Islands and wished to re-create the olfactory experience. In response her perfumer, Omar Arif, produced a scent evocative of fresh island greenery, citrus, herbs, tobacco and leather. The result was Cabochard, the essence of the Spice Islands.

Introduced   1959
Reintroduced   1972
Price   Mid-range

CABOTINE

Scent Type
Floral - Green

Composition
Top Notes: Orange blossom, tangerine, ylang-ylang, peach, plum, greens, cassie, coriander
Heart Notes: Ginger lily, iris, hyacinth, tuberose, rose, carnation, jasmine, heliotrope
Base Notes: Sandalwood, black currant bud, musk, vanilla, amber, cedarwood, civet, vetiver, tonka bean

From the House of Grès, Cabotine is a green floral harmony with dominant notes of ginger and ginger lily. Delicate florals are balanced with fruity top notes and sensual spicy base notes. Subtle, fresh and long-lasting.

The exquisite bottle is wreathed with frosted emerald glass flowers and topped with a similar green floral stopper echoing the green fragrance notes. A beautiful flacon, it is destined to be a collector's item. Other products in Cabotine are powder, lotion, gel and soap.

Wonder what the name means? Cabotine is French for "mischief."

Introduced   1990
Price   Mid-range

CAESARS WOMAN

Scent Type
Floral - Ambery

Composition
> *Top Notes:* *Orange blossom, geranium*
> *Heart Notes:* *Egyptian jasmine, rose, iris*
> *Base Notes:* *Tibetan musk, sandalwood, patchouli*

Famous Patrons
> *Carol Channing*

From Caesars Merchandising for the renowned Caesars Palace hotel and casino comes Caesars Woman, an exotic spicy floral that rests on a bed of precious woods. Introduced by the team of Jim Roth and David Horner, who helped bring the world Giorgio, Caesars Woman is a dramatic, long-lasting scent, designed to evoke the carefree privileged life in ancient Rome. Ideal for alluring days and opulent evenings.

The fragrance was launched at a celebrity-packed gala that included George Burns, Carol Channing, and models clad as Roman gladiators. Henry Gluck, Caesars chairman of the board, says, "Like everything else we do, we have been careful to create a product which bears the elegance and style associated with our resorts."

Caesars says the fragrance bottle is a " derivative of Lalique and Baccarat styles, imported from France." The scent is packaged in a rich marbleized box, accented with black and gold-colored Roman motifs.

Glamorous. Sexy. As the company states, "The most sensuous fragrance since Caesar invented pleasure." Available in lavish bath and body products, too. Let the games begin....

Introduced   1987
Price   *Mid-range*

CALANDRE

Scent Type
> *Floral - Aldehyde*

Composition
> *Top Notes:* *Greens, aldehydes, bergamot*
> *Heart Notes:* *Rose, jasmine, lily of the valley, geranium, orris*
> *Base Notes:* *Sandalwood, vetiver, oakmoss, amber, musk*

Famous Patrons
> *Barbara Bush*

Calandre is a classic fragrance from Spanish designer Paco Rabanne, who has dressed stars such as Jane Fonda and Raquel Welch. Barcelona native and Compar president Dr. Fernando Aleu brought together the magic of Paco Rabanne and the Puig family fragrance company to create Calandre. The fragrance is a floral blend with cool greens and mossy woods, fresh, clean and casual. When it was introduced, it was a shocking departure from heavy, sweet, sensual fragrances of the past, ushering in a new age of fresh, natural scents.

Calandre is French for "the grille of a car" and is intended to signify the modern woman's mobility. Rabanne explains: "Women today are on the move, traveling near and far to pursue careers of every endeavor. What could be a better symbol of this than the grille of a car?" Of a Ford Model-T, to be exact. This theme is carried through to the bottle, a sleek, modern design of glass and chrome from the talented team of Paco Rabanne and Pierre Dinand. The

COQUETTE

Scent Type
Oriental
Composition
Notes: *Balsamics, amber, vanillin, woods*

Famous Patrons
Socialite heiress Celia Lipton Farris

William Owen, perfumer to royalty, spices up the world with a flirtatious fragrance, Coquette. This 1994 introduction is an inviting Oriental blend, made naturally from warm, glowing balsamic aromatics with soft, sparkling undertones of amber and woods. The delightful result is subtle, yet tenacious...a smooth blend that can be worn to charm all evening.

From the French, a coquette is a woman who trifles with love, who deals with men playfully to attract amorous attention, who is stylish, often a clothes horse; a flirt of the first degree. Old movie buffs may remember a different coquette—America's sweetheart, Mary Pickford, won a 1929 Academy Award for her starring role in the talkie, *Coquette*.

Introduced	*1994*
Price	*Mid- to Top range*

CORIANDRE

Scent Type
Chypre - Floral
Composition
Top Notes: *Coriander, aldehydes, orange blossom, angelica*
Heart Notes: *Rose, geranium, lily, jasmine, orris*
Base Notes: *Sandalwood, vetiver, musk, oakmoss, patchouli*

A classic French fragrance from Jean Couturier, Coriandre is an enchanting blend of rich rosy florals, warm woods and sultry spices. Literally translated, coriander refers to a highly fragrant, sweet and slightly peppery herb of the parsley family; in Latin, *coriandrum sativum*.

The scent is also offered in body and bath products, packaged in malachite green with gold-colored accents. Reminds us of a Linda McCartney tune, "...coriander, coffee too...I'm the cook of the house...." But this is one spicy number that may keep you out of the kitchen.

Introduced	*1977*
Price	*Mid-range*

COURRÈGES IN BLUE

Scent Type
Floral
Composition
Top Notes: *French marigold, basil, bergamot, mandarin, geranium, coriander, aldehydes*
Heart Notes: *Rose, jasmine, black currant bud, peach, peony, violet, orange blossom, tuberose*
Base Notes: *Sandalwood, clove, patchouli, vetiver, cedarwood, civet, musk, amber, moss*

Courrèges in Blue is a romantic blend of rare French florals, accented by smooth, fruity top notes. The base accord is composed of exotic woods touched with spicy clove. A lovely day-to-evening fragrance.

André Courrèges apprenticed with the House of Balenciaga in the fifties before opening his own salon in Paris in 1961. He made his mark with modern collections featuring miniskirts and cosmonaut suits. Other design accomplishments include 1972 Olympic uniforms, autos, home furnishings and his own boutiques.

Introduced   1985
Price   High range

CRÉATION

Scent Type
   Chypre - Fresh
Composition
   Top Notes: Black currant bud, mango, passion fruit, peach, bergamot, lemon, mandarin, galbanum
   Heart Notes: Gardenia, jasmine, tuberose, narcissus, rose, ylang-ylang, carnation, lily of the valley
   Base Notes: Amber, oakmoss, musk, sandalwood, patchouli, vanilla, civet

The original fragrance from designer Ted Lapidus is Création, a fresh chypre that opens with citrusy bergamot and green notes. A light floral heart follows, set against a warm woody backdrop of oakmoss, amber and lingering musk.

Born in Paris in 1929, Ted Lapidus launched his women's designs in the sixties with the unisex and menswear looks. At first a men's designer, he dressed industrialists and heads of state, including President Harry Truman, then went on to suit up women such as Brigitte Bardot. Today his boutiques dot the globe, with shops in Europe, South America, North America and other points. Also look for his 1993 fragrance, Fantasme.

Introduced   1985
Price   High range

CRISTALLE

Scent Type
   Chypre - Fresh
Composition
   Top Notes: Greens, mandarin, lemon, bergamot, galbanum, basil, lavender
   Heart Notes: Rose, hyacinth, honeysuckle, jasmine, peach, lily of the valley, ylang-ylang, iris, mosses
   Base Notes: Woods, santal, musk, fruits, sandalwood, oakmoss

Cristalle is a fresh, fruity chypre blend that was originally developed as a single-strength eau de toilette to be lavished all over the body. In addition to the eau de toilette, in 1993 a new strength was introduced, the eau de parfum, a stronger, richer version with a few changes.

"A respect for one's roots and an attachment to the origins of Cristalle were the foundation of the new scent," says Jacques Polge, director of the Chanel Perfume Laboratories.

The eau de toilette version of Cristalle has a tangier top note of lemon, more citrus and brighter green herbal notes. It is a light energetic scent, perfect for sporty summertime wear. The eau de parfum is a richer composition with a few twists. Fruity mandarin replaces zesty lemon, jasmine is emphasized while greens and herbs are de-emphasized, mellow lily of the valley is added, and iris and woods are increased for new warmth and depth.

Both versions are dynamic fragrances that remind us of Mlle Chanel, whose unconstructed clothing designs were suitable for sporting activities—a radical concept in the early part of the century. These exhilarating, exuberant scents are the perfect mates to the Chanel sportswear lines of yesterday and today.

Introduced   1977
Price   Mid-range

CUIR DE RUSSIE

Scent Type
Chypre - Floral Animalic
Composition
Top Notes: Orange blossom, bergamot, mandarin, clary sage
Heart Notes: Iris, jasmine, rose, ylang-ylang, cedarwood, vetiver
Base Notes: Balsamics, leather, amber, vanilla

Cuir de Russie is a 1993 reintroduction of an elegant 1920s fragrance from Chanel. Introduced in conjunction with two other twenties scents, Gardenia and Bois des Îles, Cuir de Russie is reminiscent of a glamorous bygone era.

Cuir de Russie, or "Russian leather," is a vibrant leathery floral composition, enhanced by a lingering balsamic aura of woods, amber and vanilla. An inviting chypre classic; the perfect accent for a special evening at New York's Russian Tea Room restaurant.

At the time of writing, Cuir de Russie could be found only in the Chanel Boutiques.

Introduced   1927
Reintroduced   1993
Price   Mid-range

DELICIOUS

Scent Type
Floral
Composition
Top Notes: Narcisse, mimosa, mandarin, boronia, neroli, black currant bud
Heart Notes: Rose, jasmine, tuberose, lily of the valley, ylang-ylang, angelica
Base Notes: Sandalwood, patchouli, musk, orris

Famous Patrons
Barbara Walters
Loretta Swit
Barbra Streisand
Raquel Welch
Farah Fawcett
Shirlee (Mrs. Henry) Fonda
Jackie Collins
Jill St. John
Shakira (Mrs. Michael) Caine

Gale Hayman, creator of the original Giorgio fragrance, now brings forth Delicious, a subtle floral bouquet for the nineties.

As Gale Hayman reports: "When I tried this fragrance on my friends, they all said it was delicious. Delicious named itself. Very feminine, Beverly Hills energy, glamour, a bit sexy, yet classic and elegant at the same time." How does this uplifting floral scent compare with Giorgio? "Delicious represents the maturing of my sensibility, my sense of style," she says. "Giorgio is the energy of the eighties. Delicious is a classic, durable fragrance of the nineties, the Giorgio of our time."

Hayman worked with a French perfumer to create the scent, using almost entirely natural ingredients. Created in a subtle fashion with an opening accord of soothing fruits and gentle florals, Delicious develops an intense heart of rare flowers, including rose and jasmine, ylang-ylang and tuberose. The symphony is underscored by sensual musk and woods, and highlighted by orris, one of the most expensive and treasured ingredients in perfumery. Orris absolute is obtained from iris and has an aroma remarkably close to that of violets in bloom. The resulting composition is refined, elegant, understated, yet very long-lasting and sensual. In fact, in December, 1993, *Consumer Reports* magazine ranked it third out of sixty-six fragrances they tested for quality and integrity.

The fragrance is captured in Hayman's signature reclining leopard bottle, meant to represent sensual, powerful grace—then swathed in peach to reflect the softer scent. Enjoy Delicious for sophisticated days and alluring evenings. It is, indeed, Delicious.

While you're out shopping for Delicious, be sure to look for Gale Hayman's Youth-Lift skin care and color cosmetic line, packaged in exotic leopard spots.

Introduced	1993
Price	Mid-range

DEMI-JOUR

Scent Type
Floral

Composition
Top Notes: Bergamot, aldehydes, greens, violet
Heart Notes: Rose, orris, lily of the valley, jasmine, ylang-ylang, heliotrope
Base Notes: Musk, moss, sandalwood, cedarwood

Demi-Jour is a modern floral fragrance with a French heritage. The bouquet unfolds with a fresh green floral harmony, drying to a soft powdery wooded finish. A subtle scent, perfect for career-to-casual wear.

Demi-Jour comes from the French House of Houbigant, founded in 1775 by Jean-François Houbigant. The firm enjoyed success as a court-appointed perfumer to Napoleon III, Queen Victoria and Tsar Nicolas.

The fragrance is elegantly packaged in an old-fashioned globe of cut glass and topped with a silver-toned cap. Demi-Jour adds an enchanting sparkle to the dressing table.

Introduced	1988
Price	Top range

DESIGN

Scent Type
  Floral - Fruity
Composition
  Top Notes: Peach, orange blossom, jasmine, tuberose
  Heart Notes: Gardenia, lilac, honeysuckle, carnation
  Base Notes: Black currant bud, musk, sandalwood, civet

Famous Patrons
  Artist Sara Eyestone

Design is a white floral bouquet from Paul Sebastian. Dominant notes of orange blossom, lilac, gardenia and musk create a soft, feminine effect. A company spokesperson says Design was created to personalize itself to the wearer, drying down differently on each individual according to body chemistry. Some people may detect more florals, while others may experience a fruity aroma, or perhaps even a powdery finish.

Try Design in a variety of body and bath products.

Introduced   1986
Price   High range

DÉSIRADE

Scent Type
  Floral Semi-Oriental

Composition
  Top Notes: Italian bergamot, Russian coriander, Madagascar ylang-ylang, pineapple, aldehydes
  Heart Notes: Chinese osmanthus, jasmine, rose, cassia, tuberose, orange blossom, violet
  Base Notes: Sandalwood, patchouli, vetiver, Somalian opopanax, plum, raspberry, vanilla, musk

Désirade hails from the the Parisian firm of Parfums Aubusson. Désirade, meaning "the essence of desire," tantalizes with a vivid citrus top note enhanced by sparkling aldehydes, like a crisp crescendo. The scent unfolds, revealing rich florals backed up by a lingering aura of woods, fruits and animal oils. Désirade is an assertive, evocative blend, not for the shy of heart.

Housed in a frosted glass flacon of sculpted symmetry, Désirade is presented in hues of salmon pink and deep blue.

Introduced   1990
Price   Mid-range

DESTINY

Scent Type
  Floral - Fresh
Composition
  Notes: Calla lilies, white rose, fo-ti-tieng, osmanthus, karo karunde, white orchid, narcissus

Destiny is an ethereal floral fragrance from Marilyn Miglin of Chicago, who also offers a fine line of cosmetics and skin treatments.

Marilyn Miglin is joined in the business by her mother, Helen, and her daughter, Helena. A trio of brainy beauties, all are glamorous, sophisticated and accomplished. Destiny reflects the qualities these women share. The light, sparkling fragrance is created with pure white flowers, essences known for their "calming, energizing and aphrodisiac qualities," says Miglin. Essences of inspiration, confidence and inner harmony.

In perfumery, the fragrance strength of a flower and its color are related. The lighter the blossom, the more fragrant. Therefore, white flowers such as those used in Destiny are among the most prized for their fragrance.

Miglin speaks of her inspiration for Destiny: "I was in Switzerland in 1984 vacationing with my family. We were in a hot-air balloon slowly drifting over the Alpine mountains. The white flowers on the mountaintops portrayed a pure, beautiful and serene energy against the clear blue sky. They sparked in me a sense of awe and wonderment about being alive. I decided that there had to be a perfume that captured that ethereal quality and it should be called Destiny."

Even the bottle is designed to reflect an "upward movement of energy," says Miglin. In this vein, Miglin has established a mentorship program for women, called Women of Destiny. The women selected serve as mentors to others. She explains, "I believe the best way for women to make that journey is by helping other women achieve their destinies." For more information, contact the Marilyn Miglin offices in Chicago.

| Introduced | 1990 |
| Price | Mid-range |

DI BORGHESE

Scent Type
  Floral - Oriental
Composition
  Top Notes: *Greens, moss*
  Heart Notes: *Jasmine, hyacinth, lily of the valley, narcissus*
  Base Notes: *Amber, sandalwood, spices*

Famous Patrons
  Princess Marcella di Borghese

Di Borghese is a provocative fragrance personally created by the Princess—yes, there really is a Princess Marcella di Borghese, a member of the Italian royal family.

The fragrance unfolds with the freshness of green mosses, enhanced by a plethora of heady florals. Exotic spices, amber and sandalwood are swirled together to create a lingering warmth, ideal for sophisticated day wear.

Di Borghese is a rich, opulent scent, perfect for sultry Italian evenings...and fit for Italian royalty.

| Introduced | 1978 |
| Price | High range |

DIAMONDS AND EMERALDS

Scent Type
Floral

Composition
Top Notes: Gardenia, white rose, apricot, tangerine, peach, sage, hyacinth, orange blossom, greens
Heart Notes: Jasmine, lily of the valley, carnation, rose, tuberose, magnolia, wild lily
Base Notes: Vanilla, amber, musk, patchouli, vetiver, tonka bean

Diamonds and Emeralds is an Elizabeth Taylor fragrance from Parfums International, and is one of a trio of fragrances that borrow their names from emeralds, sapphires and rubies. As a connoisseur of precious gems, Elizabeth Taylor paired the elegance and brilliance of diamonds with other favorite gems. "Emeralds, rubies and sapphires share with diamonds the magic and mystery of being of the earth," she says, "and each woman who wears these gems adds her own magic and mystery to them. That's why this collection of fragrances had to be named for these jewels."

Emeralds are often associated with Venus, goddess of love, and regarded as a symbol of faith, immortality and rejuvenation of nature. Nature is reflected in Diamonds and Emeralds' top notes of fresh greenery, fruits and delicate white florals. The bouquet is underscored with sweet amber and vanilla, while the addition of tenacious musk and patchouli serves to extend

the fragrance. Diamonds and Emeralds is a lovely, feminine floral in the classic tradition.

The flacons are drop-dead gorgeous, as are all in the Jewel Collection. The eau de parfum is encased in a cylinder collared in shimmering *faux* and pavé stones of crystal and emerald green. The perfume is housed in a gently rounded clear flacon crowned with a magnificent emerald-colored rhinestone encrusted bow, tucked in a velvet box. Outer packaging is of the deepest emerald green.

Introduced   1993
Price   High range

DIAMONDS AND RUBIES

Scent Type
Floral - Oriental

Composition
Top Notes: Peach, red rose, Amazon lily, living French lilac, living peach, bitter almond
Heart Notes: Jasmine, cattleya orchid, heliotrope, spices, rose, ylang-ylang, wild lily of the valley
Base Notes: Amber, cedarwood, vanilla, benzoin, musk, sandalwood

Diamonds and Rubies made its debut into Elizabeth Taylor's fragrance collection in a sensual Oriental fashion. The fragrance reflects the passionate red fire of rubies, a gemstone rarer than diamonds. Many consider the ruby a symbol of fortune, luck, happiness and success, with a warmth and vibrancy that stir the soul.

Diamonds and Rubies unfolds with mellow peach and the classic scent of red roses. Florals and spices are found at the heart, backed up with a dramatic Oriental blend of woods, amber and sweet vanilla. A warm, passionate scent, beautiful for cool evenings and gala balls. We like it for chilly winter walks on the beach and Christmas in Aspen.

Diamonds and Rubies is presented in the same style packaging as Diamonds and Emeralds, but with *faux* and pavé stones of crystal and ruby tones. Outer packaging is in vibrant ruby, making it a beautiful gift for Valentine's Day or Christmas.

Introduced   1993
Price   High range

DIAMONDS AND SAPPHIRES

Scent Type
Floral - Fruity
Composition
Top Notes: *Freesia, lily of the valley, melon, peach, galbanum*
Heart Notes: *Rose, jasmine, rhubrum lily, ylang-ylang, spices, tagetes*
Base Notes: *Sandalwood, vetiver, amber, musk*

Diamonds and Sapphires rounds out the 1993 gemstone trio for Elizabeth Taylor's fragrance collection, as the sibling to Diamonds and Emeralds, and Diamonds and Rubies. (Rumor has it though, that more gemstones may be added.) Parfums International explained the selection of sapphires to represent the fragrance with a colorful illustration: "The ancients believed the world rested on a giant sapphire and that the reflection of this stone colored the entire universe from the sea to the sky." Imagine the cool ocean depths, the serene evening sky. Soothing and subtle.

The theme is carried out through fruity top notes combined with cool freesia and effervescent lily of the valley. A light floral heart gives way to a subtle woody drydown. A playful, lighthearted fragrance equally suitable for summer picnics and light office wear. Take this one to the beach...say, Acapulco or the French Riviera.

The Diamonds and Sapphires packaging is resplendent, accented with *faux* sapphire-colored rhinestones. The line is packaged in the most brilliant sapphire blue. This item goes at the top of our Hanukkah gift list.

Elizabeth Taylor is involved in all aspects of her fragrances, from development to marketing and promoting. She gives one hundred percent and is tireless in her personal appearances in department stores. Aside from her fragrance business, this brilliant actress is a dedicated activist in the fight against AIDS. From her Oscar-winning performances in *Butterfield 8* and *Who's Afraid of Virginia Woolf?* to her 1994 role in *The Flintstones* as Pearl Slaghoople (Fred's mother-in-law) to her humanitarian concerns, personal trials and business ventures, she sets an example for survival and success. Grace, strength, talent and passion.

Her devotion to philanthropic organizations is felt around the world as she lends her fundraising ability to a long list of needy causes, including UNICEF, the Variety Children's Hospital, AIDS Project Los Angeles and the American Foundation for AIDS Research. For founding the latter organization, she was honored in 1987 with France's most prestigious award, the Legion of Honor. But she didn't stop there. In 1991 she created the Elizabeth Taylor AIDS Foundation to provide patient care, prevention and research toward an AIDS cure.

She sums it all up saying: "Celebrity is not something that comes without responsibility. If I can further a worthwhile cause simply by lending my voice, I feel that it is my place do so."

Introduced   1993
Price   High range

DILYS

Scent Type
Floral
Composition
Top Notes: Orange blossom, neroli, narcissus
Heart Notes: Moroccan rose, French jasmine, tuberose, ylang-ylang, lily of the valley
Base Notes: Sandalwood, musk, oakmoss

Laura Ashley's second fragrance, after her first namesake scent, is Dilys, a subtle feminine creation.

The fragrance begins with sweet fruit notes, blending into a classic French composition of rose, jasmine and other rich florals, finally drying down to a powdery sandalwood base with touches of musk for added staying power.

The delicate bottle is wreathed with frosted flowers and wrapped in peach tones—the perfect enhancement to any woman's elegant dressing table.

Introduced   1991
Price   High range

DIONNE

Scent Type
Oriental - Ambery
Composition
Top Notes: Rose, bergamot, orange blossom
Heart Notes: Rose, jasmine, lily of the valley, patchouli, sandalwood, cedarwood
Base Notes: Moss, amber, vanilla, musk, benzoin, tonka bean

Famous Patrons
Dionne Warwick
Lyricist and singer Carol Conners
Designer Kathleen Baughman
Talent agent Joan Mangum

Singer Dionne Warwick hadn't planned on launching her own fragrance when she asked Linda Marshall, president of Elysee Scientific Cosmetics, to help her create a fragrance. "I simply wanted my own distinctive perfume," she says. Warwick and Marshall worked together to create Dionne, a scent that Marshall says is the very essence of Warwick. Next, Warwick gave samples to her close friends at her birthday party and the scent turned out to be a hit. At Christmas she surprised her friends with signed crystal flacons of her fragrance, and suddenly she found herself in the perfume business.

It's not surprising that along with her hit records she now has a hit fragrance, for she worked with the perfumer the way she creates music—combining notes to create unique fragrance chords.

The sumptuous Oriental bouquet carries an unusual top note, created from the finest floral essences. The green floral heart is enhanced by sweet mossy amber, the lingering aromatic theme.

Warwick advises lavish use of the heady fragrance: "Wearing perfume is like loving. You can't be stingy. You have to give yourself abundantly, not just a little here and there."

Introduced   *1986*
Price   *Mid-range*

DIORELLA

Scent Type
   Chypre - Fresh
Composition
   Top Notes: *Sicilian lemon, greens, basil, Italian bergamot, melon*
   Heart Notes: *Moroccan jasmine, rose, carnation, cyclamen*
   Base Notes: *Oakmoss, vetiver, musk, patchouli*

Diorella is an ethereal chypre blend from the House of Christian Dior. Diorella splashes on with cool citrus and greens, followed by radiant light florals and a mossy base note. The fragrance is a superb example of the classic citrus-moss chypre blend, so named after the Mediterranean island of Cyprus where many of the ingredients are found.

Christian Dior apprenticed in Paris at the atelier of Robert Piguet before opening his own salon in 1946. His timing was perfect, and his feminine New Look collection of swirling skirts, tiny waists and glamorous gowns became the rage in postwar Paris. Dior's classic suits set the trend in the fifties until his death in 1957. The reins then passed to a twenty-one-year-old named Yves Saint Laurent, who headed the company until 1960 when he left to serve in the Algerian war. Today the House of Dior still leads the way with artful creations in fashion and fragrance.

Introduced   *1972*
Price   *High range*

DIORESSENCE

Scent Type
   Oriental - Spicy
Composition
   Top Notes: Aldehydes, greens, fruits
   Heart Notes: Jasmine, geranium, cinnamon,
   carnation, tuberose, ylang-ylang, orris
   Base Notes: Patchouli, oakmoss, vetiver,
   benzoin, vanilla, musk, styrax

Dioressence is a sophisticated Oriental blend of florals and spices from the House of Christian Dior. A voluptuous, opulent fragrance for women of confidence. Dioressence is beautiful for cool symphony evenings under a layer of mink or cashmere.

Introduced   1980
Price   High range

DIORISSIMO

Scent Type
   Floral - Fresh
Composition
   Top Notes: Greens, bergamot, calyx
   Heart Notes: Lily of the valley, jasmine,
   boronia, rosewood, ylang-ylang, lilac
   Base Notes: Sandalwood, civet

The second fragrance (after Miss Dior) introduced by Christian Dior was Diorissimo. The dominant note is the light, ethereal essence of lily of the valley. A delicate floral—feminine, fresh, innocent and romantic. Stylish and mannered in the Dior tradition.

The serene fragrance was developed by master perfumer Edmond Roudnitska, who is said to have relied upon dreamlike springtime images to create Diorissimo. He described Diorissimo, saying, "This is a pure lily of the valley scent that also has the odor of the woods in which it is found and the indefinable atmosphere of springtime." Thus the airy, celestial quality of the fragrance. Always right, never overpowering.

Introduced   1956
Price   High range

DIVA

Scent Type
   Chypre - Floral
Composition
   Top Notes: Mandarin, ylang-ylang,
   Indian tuberose, cardamom, bergamot,
   coriander, aldehydes
   Heart Notes: Honeyed Moroccan rose,
   Turkish rose, Egyptian jasmine,
   Florentine iris, narcissus, carnation, orris
   Base Notes: Patchouli, ambergris, oakmoss,
   sandalwood, vetiver, musk, civet, honey

Diva is a rich chypre blend from high fashion designer Emanuel Ungaro. The fragrance opens with fresh fruit tones, followed by rosy floral notes underscored by exotic woods. Indulgent, romantic and sensual—a diva embodied.

Emanuel Ungaro worked under Balenciaga and Courrèges before opening his own business in Paris in 1965. Today he is known for his use of vivid color and soft fluid lines in designs that are sophisticated and elegant, as mirrored in his fragrance packaging. In fact, the Diva bottle is fashioned after an Ungaro dress, featuring soft drapes that meet in the center of the flacon.

Introduced   1983
Price   High range

DNA PERFUME
BY
BIJAN

Scent Type
Floral - Ambery
Composition
Top Notes: Rosewood, minty geranium, ylang-ylang, bergamot
Heart Notes: Jasmine, lily of the valley, tuberose, clove, osmanthus
Base Notes: Myrrh, oakmoss, sandalwood, vetiver, vanilla, benzoin, amber

DNA Perfume is the creation of internationally celebrated designer Bijan. DNA incorporates the initials of his children, Daniela, Nicolas and Alexandra. Certainly gene-inspired. Bijan states, "I think in the nineties, the sexy type of attitude is about reality and family." His DNA ads feature his beautiful wife, Tracy, with Alexandra and Nicolas.

DNA Perfume, which the company describes as a "floramber naturelle," begins with the mellowness of rosewood, quickly followed by tangy bergamot and geranium. The fragrance evolves to a feminine floral bouquet resting amidst a subtle earthy blend of greens, spices and amber. A soft, romantic and sensual fragrance that ultimately responds to—what else?—your personal deoxyribonucleic acid, or DNA.

The fragrance is packaged in a bottle shaped like intertwined spiral strands of DNA. Bijan enthuses: "Our senses remind us we are alive. Celebrate!"

Introduced   1993
Price   Top range

DOLCE & GABBANA

Scent Type
Floral - Oriental
Composition
Top Notes: Tangerine, basil, ivy, freesia, petitgrain
Heart Notes: Bulgarian rose, marigold, lily of the valley, orange blossom, red carnation, jasmine, coriander
Base Notes: Sandalwood, tonka bean, vanilla, musk

The signature fragrance from the fiery, dynamic Italian design team, Domenico Dolce and Stefano Gabbana. Dolce & Gabbana is a smooth floral Oriental blend, with spirited top notes of tangerine and freesia. It was honored with the 1993 International Award from the Italian Accademia del Profumo for best women's fragrance.

In the United States, the fragrance was initially launched exclusively at Neiman Marcus. Reportedly, Dolce and Gabbana had a hand in the overall package design, a composition in hues of deep ruby red and velvety gold. The bottle is a study in right angles, from the rectangular glass flask to the gold-colored collar and crowning stopper. Finally, the entire ensemble is swathed in red velvet.

Dolce and Gabbana designs are attracting the attention of some of the world's most interesting women. Isabella Rossellini and Sherilyn Fenn happily agreed to appear in Dolce and Gabbana ads, while Madonna rang them for help with her 1993-94 *Girlie Show* tour costumes. Dolce and Gabbana complied, and Madonna and her dancers pranced through the show wearing many of their designs.

Dolce and Gabbana say they created the scent with strong-willed women in mind and that they drew their inspiration from Italian actresses Sophia Loren, Gina Lollobrigida and Anna Magnani. Beautiful, strong-willed women indeed.

Introduced	*1993*
Price	*Top range*

DONNA KARAN
NEW YORK

Scent Type
Floral

Composition
Top Notes: *Casablanca lily, apricot*
Heart Notes: *Rose, cassia, ylang-ylang, jasmine, heliotrope*
Base Notes: *Suede, amber, sandalwood, patchouli*

Leading trade magazine *Beauty Fashion* reports that this signature scent is based on a few of Donna Karan's favorite things: "Casablanca lilies, the warmth of cashmere, and the skin scent of suede." The fragrance was born of a three-year collaboration between Karan and her husband. She calls it a sexy day-to-evening scent, designed for subtle sophistication. The predominantly floral composition is accented by soft Oriental chypre notes of leathery suede, amber and patchouli.

Karan's husband and business partner, artist-sculptor Stephen Weiss, designed the black bottle that is destined to be a collector's item. The swirls reflect the graceful silhouette of a woman's form, and hand-painted 24-karat gold accents match the gold-colored tea paper packaging. Weiss says, "The bottle is a gift to my wife, to women, to today and to life."

The fragrance is available through the Donna Karan Beauty Company and DKNY boutiques, and in hundreds of fine department stores. The fragrance is a lovely addition to her line of clothing and accessories.

Introduced	*1992*
Price	*Top range*

DUNE

Scent Type
Floral - Oceanic
Composition
Floral Notes: *Lily, wallflower, peony*
Oceanic Notes: *Amber, broom, lichen*

Dune hails from the house of acclaimed French couturier Christian Dior. It was honored in 1993 with a FiFi Award, in the category of Women's Fragrance of the Year in Limited Distribution. Dior describes Dune as a floral oceanic blend, creating a new olfactory category. The effect is fresh and natural, ideal for summer, daytime, sports or anytime a light soothing scent is desired.

The House of Dior says Dune is "the perfume of serenity [that] tells the story of woman and nature intermingled...a place for serenity, meditation, and harmony." A haven from stress, Dune is described as an understated composition with natural roots, like flowers strewn on the sand. Dior donated $350,000 to the Nature Conservatory Foundation, for its "Protect the Dunes" program.

The fragrant concoction is housed in a fluid apricot-hued flacon tucked inside a box of Persian orange, the color of the sun setting over sand dunes.

Introduced 1992
Price *Mid-range*

EARTHSOURCE

A collection of three fragrances.

RAINSWEPT JASMINE

Scent Type
Floral - Fresh
Composition
Top and Heart Notes: *Jasmine, freesia, lily of the valley, hyacinth, melon*
Base Notes: *Musk, sandalwood*

SUNWARMED PEACH

Scent Type
Floral - Fruity
Composition
Top and Heart Notes: *Peach, lily of the valley, rose, violet, ylang-ylang*
Base Notes: *Oakmoss, patchouli*

WINDFRESH FLOWERS

Scent Type
Floral
Composition
Top and Heart Notes: *Amazon lily, rose, jonquil, mimosa*
Base Notes: *Tree moss, musk, sandalwood*

The EarthSource scents are naturally rich fragrances formed from essences found in nature: botanicals, herbs and spices. Each is available in a complete line of body care products, as well as home environment products, such as potpourri, candles and incense.

EarthSource is an environmentally friendly line: All packaging is made from recycled or recyclable materials. Products are not animal tested or animal derived. In keeping with this philosophy, for the launch each EarthSource product was packed with a Plant-A-Tree coupon. When the coupon was returned, a tree was planted in each person's name in coordination with Global ReLeaf and the American Forests. An imaginative way to launch a fragrance and a forest. Now the fun part: After returning the coupon, each person received a "Sappy Birch Announcement." Ours informed us that a tree had been planted in the H. Alpert Heritage Forest in the Kettle Moraine State Park, Wisconsin. Our offspring weighed two ounces, measured three inches tall, and was in excellent health with a full head of green hair.

The moderately priced line is perfect for warm weather and casual daytime wear. A delightful collection of youthful, spirited fragrances.

Introduced   1992
Price   Mid-range

EAU D'HADRIEN

Scent Type
  Chypre - Fresh

Composition
  Notes: *Sicilian lemon, grapefruit, citron, cypress*

Eau d'Hadrien is crisp and tart, refreshing and refined, a fragrance that can be worn by women and men. The vibrant scent from Annick Goutal is available in a light eau de toilette, as well as a more concentrated eau de toilette. It is a zesty scent, perfect for daytime and sporty active wear.

Eau d'Hadrien is Goutal's personal morning scent, the fresh fragrance she splashes on and wears at home in the early hours. As the day progresses, she recommends layering other fragrances from her collection right over it. In fact, the entire Goutal line is made to be mixed and layered for unique interpretations.

Introduced   1986
Price   High range

EAU D'HERMÈS

Scent Type
  Floral - Fruity
Composition
  Top Notes: *Cardamom, herbal lavender, petitgrain lemon, cinnamon, cumin*
  Heart Notes: *Jasmine, Bourbon geranium, vanilla, tonka bean, labdanum*
  Base Notes: *Sandalwood, cedarwood, flamed birch*

Eau d'Hermès is a noble fragrance created by master perfumer Edward Roudnitska. A celestial blend of florals and fruits, enhanced with a touch of spice. It was recently relaunched on the 150th anniversary of the House of Hermès.

Look for Eau d'Hermès at Hermès specialty stores.

Introduced   1951
Price   Top range

EAU DE CAMILLE

Scent Type
　　Floral - Green
Composition
　　Notes: Honeysuckle, ivy, grass, seringa

Created by Renaissance woman Annick Goutal—former concert pianist and model, now an accomplished perfumer.

This fragrance was named in honor of her daughter, Camille. One day her daughter opened a window in their home in France, and Goutal was inspired by the scents wafting through, the smell of ivy and vines and fresh-cut grass, of honeysuckle and other fresh florals. This spirited green floral is available in a light eau de toilette and a concentrated eau de toilette.

For a true delight, visit Goutal's store on the rue de Castiglione in Paris' elegant Seventh *Arrondissement.* Her private laboratory is upstairs, where she creates her fragrant world with ingredients from the perfume mecca of

Grasse, France. She also has a line of men's fragrances, bath and beauty products, skin care and home fragrances.

Annick Goutal says of her creative endeavor: "Nature and all her wonders guide me....Emotions find expression in fragrance. Fragrance is the music of my dreams. Fragrance is my inspiration."

Introduced   1986
Price   High range

EAU DE CHARLOTTE

Scent Type
　　Floral - Fruity
Composition
　　Notes: Mimosa, black currant bud, cocoa, lily of the valley

A warm, mellow blend of fruits and florals, Eau de Charlotte is a delightful, easy-to-wear fragrance, available in several strengths.

Eau de Charlotte is packaged in curved, ribbed glass flacons crowned with gold-colored caps. The concentrated eau de toilette and perfumes are housed in rounded opaque bottles, topped with Annick Goutal's signature golden butterfly. For women on the go, some natural sprays and butterfly bottles are presented in a gold lamé purse. Outer packaging for all of her fragrances is in hues of ivory and gold.

Introduced   1986
Price   High range

EAU DE COLOGNE DU COQ

Scent Type
Citrus
Composition
Top Notes: Hesperides, lemon, bergamot, neroli
Heart Notes: Lavender, jasmine, patchouli
Base Notes: Moss, sandalwood

A fragrance from the founder of the Guerlain empire, Jacques Guerlain. This century-old classic is a dry, crisp citrus splash. It is available only in cologne and is packaged in the distinctive "bee bottle," a flacon created in honor of the Napoléonic court.

Eaux de cologne are often classified as "hesperides," meaning that they are made from the fruit of citrus trees. We found a romantic history behind the term, too. In Greek mythology, Hesperides were garden nymphs who guarded the wedding gift of golden apples from Gaea to Hera. Hesperia was also the ancient Greek name for Italy and the Roman name for Spain.

Most of these hesperides, or citrus eaux de cologne, are worn by both sexes. They are perfect for sporty active wear, hot humid days, or high-pressure offices.

Introduced 1894
Price Mid-range

EAU DE COLOGNE HERMÈS

Scent Type
Citrus
Composition
Top Notes: Mint, mango, papaya, buchu bark, lemon, mandarin, bergamot, basil, coriander
Heart Notes: Neroli, orange leaves, lily of the valley, honeysuckle, lavender, rosemary
Base Notes: Petitgrain citron, oakmoss, patchouli, musk, cedarwood, sandalwood

Another classic fragrance from Hermès Paris, Eau de Cologne Hermès is a fresh, invigorating blend suitable for men and women. The bright accords of citrus and mint are ideal for daytime, summer, active wear—anytime a fresh, clean scent is preferred. Perhaps right after a sunrise canter on your trusty horse with the Hermès saddle, your favorite silk Hermès scarf flying in the breeze behind you. Ah...we live for luxuries. The scent dries down to subtle notes of woods and greens, ideal for natural, relaxed wear.

Eau de Cologne is available in an array of products, from shampoo to cremes to soap and deodorant. Look for the fragrance in the vivid signature green bottle and the orange package.

Introduced 1979
Price Mid-range

EAU DE COLOGNE IMPÉRIALE

Scent Type
  Citrus
Composition
  Top Notes: *Hesperides, orange blossom, bergamot, neroli, lemon*
  Heart Notes: *Lavender*
  Base Notes: *Rosemary, tonka bean, cedarwood*

Famous Patrons
  Empress Eugénie

Eau de Cologne Impériale is a timeless, invigorating citrus scent that has been used by men and women for well over a century. The citrus blend is lightened with orange blossom and minty rosemary. A stimulating, subtle blend, it can be worn anytime.

As the name suggests, Eau de Cologne Impériale is a fragrance of royalty. Master perfumer Pierre-François-Pascal Guerlain, the founder of the House of Guerlain, created the fragrance for the Empress Eugénie and placed it in a flacon known as the "bee bottle" to honor the Empire, because the bee was a symbol of the Royal Court and of the industriousness of the Second Napoléonic Empire. Today, the French imperial crest is still prominently displayed on the bee bottle.

Empress Eugénie was born in Spain and became the wife of the second Louis Napoléon, also known as Napoléon III. Noted for her beauty, she favored fragrances from the House of Guerlain and gowns from the House of Worth. Due to her patronage and enjoyment of fine fragrances, the House of Guerlain made rapid advances among its well-to-do clientele. Eau de Cologne Impériale remains one of the most enduring fragrances of our time. It is available in cologne and eau de toilette.

Introduced   1853
Price   Mid-range

EAU DE GIVENCHY

Scent Type
  Floral - Fruity
Composition
  Top Notes: *Bergamot, spearmint, tagetes, greens, fruits*
  Heart Notes: *Jasmine, lily of the valley, rose, cyclamen, orris*
  Base Notes: *Musk, cedarwood, sandalwood, moss*

Eau de Givenchy is a light, fresh floral created by the House of Givenchy for a youthful clientele. The mild floral bouquet is accented with greens and fruits. Available only in an eau de toilette, it is perfect for active summer days and nights.

Hubert de Givenchy was just twenty-five years old when he opened his own couture salon in Paris 1952. His clean, youthful lines garnered immediate praise. Today, the House of Givenchy continues its women's couture, along with fragrance, ready-to-wear, menswear, accessories and other innovative ideas.

Introduced   1987
Price   *Mid-range*

EAU DE GUCCI

Scent Type
  Floral - Fresh
Composition
  Top Notes: *Mandarin, ylang-ylang, greens,*
  bergamot, hyacinth, lemon
  Heart Notes: *Jasmine, lilac, lily of the valley,*
  honeysuckle, orris, tuberose, rose
  Base Notes: *Cedarwood, amber, musk,*
  vetiver, moss, sandalwood

This light fragrance from the Italian fashion House of Gucci is a delicate floral with a soft powdery wooded base. It is ideal for sports and active summer wear, and attractively priced for a couture fragrance.

The House of Gucci was established at the beginning of the twentieth century by Guccio Gucci in Italy. Later joined by his three sons, Gucci set a high standard for leather saddles, shoes and bags. Today a wide selection of products bear the Gucci emblem.

Introduced   1984
Price   *Mid-range*

EAU DE GUERLAIN

Scent Type
  Citrus
Composition
  Top Notes: *Lemon, bergamot, basil,*
  petitgrain, fruits, caraway
  Heart Notes *Thyme, mint, lavender,*
  jasmine, carnation, patchouli, rose,
  sandalwood
  Base Notes: *Moss, amber, musk*

Eau de Guerlain is a fresh, sparkling *eau fraîche* composed by Jean-Paul Guerlain, an invigorating scent worn by women and men.

In eighteenth-century England, the Victorians assigned meaning to flowers, herbs and plants. While some of these terms are merely romantic, others are quite fitting. For example, in the Victorian language of flowers, lemon blossoms signify zest, and thyme is the symbol of activity, an appropriate description for this herb with its pine-like vigor. Eau de Guerlain, with dominant notes of lemon and thyme, mint and lavender, is a modern, sporty scent, fresh and stimulating. It is available in only one strength, the eau de toilette.

Introduced   1974
Price   *Mid-range*

EAU DE PATOU

Scent Type
  Citrus

Composition
> **Top Notes:** *Sicilian citron, Guinea oranges, Grasse petitgrain*
> **Heart Notes:** *Tunisian orange blossom, pepper, nasturtium, honeysuckle, ylang-ylang*
> **Base Notes:** *Musk, moss, amber, civet, labdanum*

From the French company of Jean Patou comes a crisp citrus scent that is perfect to splash on before a heated game of tennis or a hot business deal. An eau de cologne that is enjoyed by both sexes, it features juicy top notes balanced by a fresh floral heart and cool drydown notes.

Look for it packaged in ringed frosted glass flacons with sporty accents of marine blue and white, ready to pack for your next ocean voyage. Yachting, anyone?

Introduced	*1976*
Price	*Mid-range*

EAU DE ROCHAS

Scent Type
> *Chypre - Fresh*

Composition
> **Top Notes:** *Sicilian lime, Calabrian mandarin, bergamot, tangerine, grapefruit*
> **Heart Notes:** *Wild rose, mountain narcissus*
> **Base Notes:** *Mysore sandalwood, Croatian oakmoss, amber*

Eau de Rochas is a refreshing eau de cologne from the House of Rochas. An earthy natural, the cool chypre scent begins with tangy citrus notes, often called hesperides, tangy and uplifting. A floral heart adds depth, while woods, oakmoss and amber combine to create a lingering aura of deep green forest.

The bottle is shaped like rock crystal and nestled in a box clothed with the cool colors of a fast-running stream—images reflective of the shimmering fragrance.

Introduced	*1970*
Price	*Mid-range*

EAU DU CIEL

Scent Type
> *Floral*

Composition
> **Notes:** *Brazilian rosewood, iris, violet*

Eau du Ciel derives its name from French for "sky" or "heaven." Annick Goutal created this tender scent, christening it "a hymn to balmy summer days recalling the special delights of childhood." Ah, we can almost smell it now.... At the time of writing, Eau du Ciel was available only in a light eau de toilette.

Annick Goutal aids her olfactory memory with a notebook in which she records thousands of fragrance combinations, along with her personal associations, such as "the candies in the green bakery," or "the dunes on the Ile de Ré," one of her favorite vacation spots. The latter became the basis for a scent she created for her husband, Sables, to which she added a dash of bergamot and sandalwood.

The world is indeed a sweeter-smelling place thanks to the artistry of Annick Goutal.

Introduced   1986
Price   High range

EAU FRAÎCHE BY LÉONARD

Scent Type
Citrus
Composition
Top Notes: *Italian bergamot, mandarin, Sicilian lemon*
Heart Notes: *Florals, clove, coriander*
Base Notes: *Haitian vetiver, Singapore patchouli*

Eau Fraîche is a refreshing citrus blend from Léonard Parfums that may be used by women or men. Sparkling essence of lemon, mandarin and bergamot is supported by a soft backdrop of florals, spices and woods. Perfect for daytime, après spa or in warm weather—anytime a fresh, light fragrance is desired. In fact, Eau Fraîche in French means "cool, fresh water."

Introduced   1974
Price   Mid-range

ECCO

Scent Type
Floral
Composition
Top Notes: *Rose*
Heart Notes: *Jasmine, magnolia*
Base Notes: *Civet, musk*

Another fragrance from royal Italian entrepreneur Princess Marcella di Borghese is the romantic Ecco, a feminine, classic blend of rose and jasmine that is enhanced by a long-lasting base of civet and musk. In fact, rose and musk were favorite scents of another woman of royalty, the Empress Josephine of France, wife of Napoléon I.

Musk is a strong fixative that blends well with floral bouquets—so strong that Arab mosques built more than a thousand years ago with mortar containing musk still retain the odor.

Ecco roughly translates from Italian as "living for the moment—right here, right now." Enjoy Ecco, in the luxury of today.

Introduced   1960
Price   Mid-range

ELIZABETH TAYLOR'S PASSION

Scent Type
Floral Semi-Oriental

Composition
> **Top Notes:** *Gardenia, jasmine, lily of the valley, ylang-ylang, rose*
> **Heart Notes:** *Spices, musk*
> **Base Notes:** *Indian patchouli, Indian sandalwood, incense, cedarwood, moss*

Passion was the first fragrance from one of the best-loved actresses of all time. A feminine formula of white flowers and spicy, exotic base notes produces a very wearable, memorable scent; a fragrance for passionate living.

Elizabeth Taylor was personally involved in the creation of the Parfums International scent and describes Passion saying: "It has a scent of mystery, slightly effusive, kind of smoky and sweet. There is ylang-ylang in it, which gives it a wonderful hint of tangy, crisp freshness, and lilies of the valley...brides use this in bouquets, that's probably why I'm so attracted to it!"

What inspired the name Passion? "Passion is not just a word that indicates lovemaking or lust," she explains. "I think it's passion that's made me a survivor. If you care about other people, it becomes a passion. If you can reach a natural high that is bliss...that's passion. I have a passion for life and loving."

Passion is packaged in an elegantly styled diamond-faceted flacon with a plunging "V" neckline, cast in the violet shade of Taylor's magnificent eyes, and accented with gold-colored highlights. A striking addition to any dressing table.

Introduced	*1987*
Price	*Mid-range*

ELLEN TRACY

Scent Type
> *Floral*

Composition
> **Top Notes:** *Peach, galbanum, living osmanthus, living hyacinth*
> **Heart Notes:** *Jasmine, tuberose, rose, ylang-ylang*
> **Base Notes:** *Sandalwood, moss, amber*

Designer Linda Allard created a spirited modern floral for the Ellen Tracy line and Revlon. The crisp melange is introduced by fruity notes, followed by a classic floral bouquet set against a sweet backdrop of sandalwood and amber. It is the perfect touch to accessorize Ellen Tracy clothing.

The bottles are designed to look like smooth pebbles found on river banks. The line is cloaked in sophisticated hues of gray, ivory and gold.

Introduced	*1992*
Price	*High range*

ELYSIUM

Scent Type
> *Floral - Fruity*

Composition

    Top Notes: Jasmine, honeydew, ylang-ylang, dewberry, linden blossom

    Heart Notes: Lily of the valley, freesia, rose, osmanthus

    Base Notes: Sandalwood, papaya, musk, cedarwood

From the French firm of Clarins is Elysium, a delicate fruity floral concoction. In keeping with the Clarins philosophy, the scent is said to be "a celebration of the gifts of nature at their purest."

The frosted glass bottle appears windswept, with undulating waves cascading from the stopper to the base.

A nature-inspired, easy-to-wear fresh scent. At the time of this writing, it is available only in an eau de toilette and a body lotion.

Introduced	1993
Price	Mid-range

EMPREINTE

Scent Type

    Chypre - Floral Animalic

Composition

    Top Notes: Peach, bergamot, coriander, artemisia, aldehydes

    Heart Notes: Bulgarian rose, Grasse jasmine, melon, orris

    Base Notes: Amber, patchouli, oakmoss, cedarwood, sandalwood, castoreum

Meaning "imprint, or impression" in French, Empreinte is a chypre floral blend with the tang of fruity top notes, a floral heart and warm woody base notes. The lingering impression of Empreinte is leather. This first fragrance from French couturier André Courrèges moves with ease from the riding stables to the ballroom floor to a late night club. Versatile and refined.

Introduced	1970
Price	Mid-range

ENIGMA

Scent Type

    Chypre

Composition

    Top Notes: Aldehydes, greens, bergamot, coriander, pimento, herbs

    Heart Notes: Jasmine, rose, carnation

    Base Notes: Amber, woods, spices, patchouli, oakmoss

Enigma is a warm, sophisticated fragrance from Alexandra de Markoff. The smooth chypre blend is introduced by crisp aldehydes, greens and citrus, then slips into woody herbal notes. Sweet amber and patchouli complete the sensual aroma. The inviting Enigma is also available in perfumed body powder and lotion.

Introduced	1972
Price	Mid-range

ESCADA
BY
MARGARETHA LEY

Scent Type
Floral - Oriental
Composition
Top Notes: *Bergamot, hyacinth,*
peach, coconut
Heart Notes: *Orange blossom, jasmine,*
iris, carnation, frangipani flower
Base Notes: *Vanilla, musk, sandalwood*

Escada is the signature fragrance developed by the late Margaretha Ley, the supremely elegant international fashion designer from Sweden, widely noted for her inspirational use of vibrant color.

Escada borrowed its name from a champion Thoroughbred whose name is Portuguese for "staircase." With top notes of fresh, fruity florals, the scent is versatile enough to be worn during the day, yet sophisticated enough for the evening.

Two years in the making, the complex scent from Margaretha Ley and husband Wolfgang is presented in classic Escada design: a voluptuous sculpted glass heart, topped with gold-colored filigree swirls, nestled in Escada red packaging. The scent won a FiFi Award bestowed by The Fragrance Foundation.

New from Escada: seasonal fragrances. Once a year, a new scent is to be introduced with the company's current Spring/Summer theme. The special eau de toilette will be available from April through September of each year, for the season only. The heart-shaped bottle will remain the same, but watch for it in different finishes and colors, such as 1993's frosted Chiffon Sorbet in delicate hues of yellow and blue. Of course, Escada's original fragrance in the signature red heart is a mainstay, available year round. Also try the Resort body care collection, nourishing treatments packed with botanicals, herbs and organic extracts, packaged in brilliant hues.

Escada—let it capture your heart.

Introduced	*1990*
Price	*High range*

ESCAPE

Scent Type
Floral - Fruity
Composition
Top Notes: *Mandarin, apple, black currant bud, chamomile, apricot, melon, peach, plum*
Heart Notes: *Jasmine, rose, coriander, clove, carnation*
Base Notes: *Sandalwood, musk, cedarwood, oakmoss, amber*

American designer Calvin Klein compels us to travel, to get away from it all, with his fragrance Escape.

The fruity floral begins with a twist of apple, chamomile and black currant bud, then gives way to a spiced floral bouquet enveloped in lasting sandalwood and musk. Easy to wear, perfect for light daytime enjoyment.

The bottle looks as though it will slip comfortably into your suitcase. It was inspired by an antique perfume bottle and comes with a silver-hinged flip-top cap. It travels suited in green moire and parchment. As long as you're packing, slip in the Escape body and bath products—full of vitamins, minerals and deep-sea botanicals.

Escape...oh yes...just a moment, the valise is almost packed...one-way ticket please...somewhere with a deserted beach...and toned, muscled men...

Introduced   1991
Price   Mid-Range

E S T É E

Scent Type
Floral
Composition
Top Notes: Peach, raspberry, citrus oils
Heart Notes: Rose, lily of the valley, jasmine, carnation, ylang-ylang, honey, orris
Base Notes: Cedarwood, musk, moss, sandalwood, styrax

Famous Patrons
Nancy Reagan
Pat Buckley
Duchess of Windsor

Estée Lauder's namesake fragrance is a sparkling floral composition for the confident woman. Versatile and sophisticated.

Ethereal aldehydic fruity top notes are balanced with sweet florals and a finale of powdery woods and sensual musk. A fragrance as memorable as the famous women who wear it.

Introduced   1968
Price   Mid-range

E T E R N I T Y

Scent Type
Floral - Fresh
Composition
Top Notes: Mandarin, freesia, sage
Heart Notes: Narcissus, lily of the valley, marigold, white lily, jasmine, rose
Base Notes: Sandalwood, patchouli, amber, musk

The second fragrance in the string of bestsellers from Calvin Klein, Eternity is a blend of sweet white florals, topped with the fresh citrus note of mandarin, and warmed by Oriental base or background essences of sweet woods and amber. A fresh casual fragrance, equally suitable for a busy career day or a leisurely bike ride on a sunny beach.

Eternity is also available in a luxurious array of lotions, powders and cremes. Packaged in classic white.

Introduced   1988
Price   Mid-range

EVELYN

Scent Type
Floral

Composition
Top Notes: *Roses*
Heart Notes: *Rose, lily of the valley, peach*
Base Notes: *Woods, musk*

Evelyn is the first eau de parfum from Crabtree & Evelyn. The company describes the fragrance as "sophisticated and refreshing." The composition was developed around a multitude of roses. Though the singular impression is of roses, more than eighty-five ingredients were blended to achieve this effect.

Expert rose grower David Austin of Wolverhampton, England, toiled over the fragrance for eight years with master perfumer V. Mane of Grasse, France. Together they employed new "headspace technology" to exactly re-create the scent of Evelyn roses. The result—superb.

The pink liquid is showcased in a clear flacon inspired by nineteenth-century dressing table bottles. A silver cap sets off the romantic creation.

Evelyn is available at Crabtree & Evelyn stores and in select department stores.

Introduced	*1993*
Price	*Mid-range*

FAROUCHE

Scent Type
Floral - Aldehyde

Composition
Top Notes: *Bergamot, mandarin, galbanum, aldehydes, peach*
Heart Notes: *Rose, jasmine, honeysuckle, clary sage, cardamom, genista flowers, iris, carnation, geranium, lily of the valley, lily*
Base Notes: *Oakmoss, sandalwood, amber, vetiver, musk*

Farouche is an aldehydic floral bouquet from Nina Ricci. Citrus fruit top notes combine with the greenness of galbanum for a crisp opening sequence of aromas, dissolving into an ethereal floral heart. Soft sandalwood and soothing oakmoss lend a woody backdrop, like an autumn walk through the Black Forest.

Softly tenacious, a feminine fragrance that is easy to wear from day to evening for a variety of occasions.

Introduced	*1974*
Price	*High range*

FEMINITÉ DU BOIS

Scent Type
Chypre

Composition
   Top Notes: *Cedarwood, orange blossom,*
peach, honey, plum, beeswax
   Heart Notes: *Cedarwood, clove, cardamom,*
cinnamon
   Base Notes: *Cedarwood, musk*

From the Japanese cosmetic and treatment line Shiseido comes a woody fragrance with a dominant cedarwood note. The scent is formulated so that cedarwood lingers throughout, from the top note, through the heart, to the base note. Fruits and spices round out the long-lasting feminine fragrance. Close your eyes and you'll imagine you're in an evergreen forest or, if you're an urban dweller, perhaps a Christmas tree lot. Feminité du Bois is a distinctive scent for those who like a poignant earthy fragrance.

Serge Lutens was charged with the creation of Feminité du Bois. Bois is French for "woods," and Lutens was reportedly inspired by the atlas cedarwood found in Morocco, where he resides six months of every year. The fragrance was introduced at the Paris Museum of Modern Art, where fountains bubbled with it.

The fluid flacon is in the shape of a woman's slender silhouette, bathed in shades of cocoa mauve. The scent is also available in a L'Eau Timide, a lighter version with moisturizers.

Shiseido has other wooded fragrances that, at the time of this writing, are only available at the Salons du Palais Royal Shiseido in Paris. Rose de Nuit is a blend of chypre, Turkish rose, amber and musk notes. Ambre Sultan is an ambergris-based fragrance suitable for women and men. Perhaps we'll see them soon in our neighborhood.

Introduced   *1992*
Price   *High range*

FEMME

Scent Type
   Chypre - Fruity
Composition
   Top Notes: *Peach, plum, bergamot,*
lemon, rosewood
   Heart Notes: *Ylang-ylang, jasmine,*
May rose, clove, orris
   Base Notes: *Musk, amber, oakmoss,*
vanilla, patchouli, benzoin, leather

Famous Patrons
   Mae West

Femme is a full-bodied fragrance from Parfums Rochas, a fragrance as rich in history as in scent. The distinctive composition was created for the House of Rochas during World War II by the noted perfumer Edmond Roudnitska of Cabris, France. When once asked about his olfactory gift, Roudnitska replied, "The capacity to create is essentially the ability to imagine." To the perfumer, the fragrance is a composition, as evocative as a Monet masterpiece.

Marcel Rochas opened his couture salon in Paris in 1924 and quickly became known for his broad-shouldered suits, bustiers and elaborate designs. Femme was originally available only by strict invitation. Rochas sent a letter to his clients, allowing them to purchase a limited-edition, numbered bottle. Imagine the demand he created! The next year he made Femme available to the public, and he had an instant hit.

The legendary Femme explodes with Mediterranean fruits, mingled with intoxicating floral aromas and underscored with lingering balsamics and moss. A brilliant, recognizable fragrance.

The bottle, designed by René Lalique, is a sensuously curved crystal flacon, symbolic of a woman's graceful silhouette. Reportedly, it was inspired by the voluptuous Mae West, who was a personal friend of Lalique and a valued client of Rochas. Our favorite Mae West quote is, "Between two evils, I always pick the one I never tried before."

Femme—created to embody femininity.

Introduced   1944
Price   High range

FENDI

Scent Type
Chypre - Floral
Composition
Top Notes: Bergamot, aldehydes, rosewood, fruits
Heart Notes: Jasmine, rose, ylang-ylang, geranium, carnation
Base Notes: Patchouli, musk, leather, sandalwood, cedarwood, spices, amber, vanilla

Fendi is the original signature scent from the noted Italian design firm of Fendi, known for its remarkable fashions, leather goods and household designs.

The warm, subtly blended chypre floral is housed in a sleek modern rectangular flacon from Pierre Dinand. Fendi is a harmonious fragrance with a passionate Italian heart.

Introduced   1987
Price   High range

FERRE BY FERRE

Scent Type
Floral - Fruity
Composition
Top Notes: Orange blossom, bergamot, ylang-ylang, butterbush
Heart Notes: Rose, mimosa, peach, passion fruit, violet, cassia, moss, lily of the valley
Base Notes: Vanilla, sandalwood, spices, amber, iris, vetiver, musk

From the extraordinary Italian fashion designer and architect, Gianfranco Ferre, comes a complex fragrance, a melange of Italian elegance, humor and sensuality.

The prominent notes are derived from delicate white flowers, giving it a sweet, feminine persona. It comes in a bottle telling of Ferre's architectural design, a flacon of sculpted crystal, black and gold-color, topped with a faceted crystal stopper. The scent is available in body care products, too.

Introduced   1992
Price   High range

FIAMMA

Scent Type
Floral - Oriental

Composition

Top Notes: *Rose, jasmine, heliotrope,
violet, hyacinth*
Heart Notes: *Clove, carnation*
Base Notes: *Oakmoss, sandalwood, patchouli*

Created for the adventurous woman,
Fiamma takes its name from the Italian for
"fiery, unconventional."

Fiamma opens with a tumble of florals,
while heart notes of carnation and clove impart
a spicy, saucy character. The composition dries
down with an accord of smoldering aromatic
woods, with a dominant note of sensual
patchouli.

Another classic Italian fragrance from the
Princess Marcella Borghese repertoire.

Introduced	1965
Price	Mid-range

FIDJI

Scent Type
Floral

Composition

Top Notes: *Galbanum, hyacinth,
lemon, bergamot*
Heart Notes: *Carnation, orris, ylang-ylang,
jasmine, rose*
Base Notes: *Vetiver, musk, moss, sandalwood*

Fidji was introduced by fashion designer
Guy Laroche. The fragrance borrows its name
from the Fiji Islands in the South Pacific.
Appropriately, the fragrance opens with fresh
tropical notes, evolving into a radiant floral
heart. A mild base of fragrant woods produces a
soft powdery drydown. It is a perfect fragrance for
island adventures or warm weather daydreaming.

Introduced	1966
Price	Mid-range

FIRST

Scent Type
Floral - Aldehyde

Composition

Top Notes: *Aldehydes, mandarin, black
currant bud, peach, raspberry, hyacinth*
Heart Notes: *Turkish rose, narcissus,
jasmine, lily of the valley, carnation, orchid,
tuberose, orris*
Base Notes: *Amber, tonka bean, oakmoss,
sandalwood, vetiver, musk, honey, civet*

First is a fabulous floral bouquet from
world-renowned Parisian jeweler Van Cleef &
Arpels. The aldehydic note adds a brilliant
jewel-like sparkle to the rich classic scent, a rush
of fragrance that softens into a sweet amber and
wood base.

First is housed in a lovely curved glass bottle
bearing a gold-colored pinafore inscribed with
the name, and capped with a rounded, easy-to-
grasp stopper.

Before you adorn yourself with your Van Cleef & Arpels jewels, be sure to cleanse and soften your skin with First body and bath products....Gives a whole new meaning to the concept of layering, *n'est-ce pas?*

Introduced   1976
Price   High range

FLEUR DE FLEURS

Scent Type
Floral - Aldehyde
Composition
Top Notes: *Bergamot, greens, lemon, aldehydes*
Heart Notes: *May rose, Grasse jasmine, iris, hyacinth, ylang-ylang, lily of the valley, lilac, cyclamen, magnolia*
Base Notes: *Sandalwood, civet, musk*

Fleur de Fleurs is a versatile floral scent from Nina Ricci. The essence of fruits and woods adds a velvety freshness to the delicate floral heart. A carved flower adorns a rounded Lalique flacon.

Introduced   1980
Price   Mid-range

FLEURS D'ELLE

Scent Type
Floral - Green
Composition
Top Notes: *Florals, greens*
Heart Notes: *Florals*
Base Notes: *Woods*

Famous Patrons
Mamie Eisenhower

From Nettie Rosenstein, fashion designer to former First Lady Mamie Eisenhower, comes Fleurs d'Elle. Along with Coco Chanel, Rosenstein helped launch the polished "little black dress and a fine strand of pearls" look for evening wear.

Fleurs d'Elle is one of three women's scents remaining from the Rosenstein legacy and is available in a full range of fragrance, bath and body products.

Though the North American distributor, Classic Fragrances, couldn't supply the individual fragrance notes, Fleurs d'Elle suggests a floral melange introduced by soft orange blossoms and green herbs, dissolving into ylang-ylang, gardenia, narcissus, jasmine, hyacinth and rose. Subtle and soft. Ideal for casual daytime wear, leisurely luncheons or long office days.

Introduced   1950s
Price   Mid-range

FLEURS DE ROCAILLE

Scent Type
Floral
Composition
Top Notes: *Lily of the valley, clover*
Heart Notes: *Rose, violet, lilac, jasmine, iris*
Base Notes: *Sandalwood, musk, civet*

Fleurs de Rocaille is another timeless scent from the great Parisian perfumery of Caron. It is an enduring, sublime floral blend, a classic arrangement. It was introduced in an upturned glass bottle, tied with a gold-colored ribbon beneath a crystal stopper. Sophisticated simplicity.

In addition, Fleurs de Rocaille enjoyed a recent Hollywood walk-on role in the movie *Scent of a Woman*, with Al Pacino. Pacino portrays a rough-hewn military man who has lost his sight and his will to live. At the end of the movie, when he finally decides to choose life, he meets a woman and is enchanted by her, as well as her fragrance—Fleurs de Rocaille. With one deep breath he identifies the scent, and to him it represents the captivating scent of a woman.

The power of the movies...in just one scene, an entire new generation became acquainted with the classic Fleurs de Rocaille.

Introduced   1933
Price   High range

FOLAVRIL

Scent Type
Floral - Fruity
Composition
Notes: *Jasmine, mango*

Annick Goutal's Folavril bursts with naturally fresh, exotic floral notes, smoothed with tropical mango. In French, Folavril loosely translates as "fool's folly," a fun interpretation. Perfect for casual, fun-filled day wear.

Try blending Annick Goutal fragrances to create your own interpretations. For example, you can give Folavril a crisp top note through a marriage with Goutal's citrusy chypre Eau d'Hadrien. Or warm it with the deeper notes of other Goutal favorites.

Introduced   1986
Price   High range

4711 EAU DE COLOGNE

Scent Type
Chypre - Fresh
Composition
Top Notes: *Bergamot, orange oil, lemon, basil, peach*
Heart Notes: *Bulgarian rose, jasmine, melon, lily, cyclamen*
Base Notes: *Haitian vetiver, Indian sandalwood oakmoss, patchouli, cedarwood, musk*

This is the original 4711 Eau de Cologne formula first produced in eighteenth-century Germany. Invigorating citrus top notes create a tart, stimulating scent, followed by light florals and warm, exotic woods. It is a refreshing, sporty fragrance worn by women and men. Indeed, many of the herbs used in 4711 have been used historically as external application for headaches and rejuvenation, though we can't vouch for their effectiveness.

The dominant note in 4711 is bergamot, a tangy fresh oil from a nonedible citrus fruit. Perfumers tell us the best bergamot trees in the world are in Calabria, Italy. Bergamot is often found in the top notes of fragrances, especially eaux de cologne. An excellent fixative, it is also the prime ingredient in Earl Grey tea.

The history of 4711 is as rich as the fragrance: The eighteenth-century formulation was reputedly developed by a Carthusian monk. The formula came into the hands of German businessman Ferdinand Muelhens, who began marketing the cologne. When the French descended upon Germany in that century, they renumbered street addresses. The businessman found himself with a new address, Glockengasse No. 4711, Köln, a number he adopted for the cologne. The name and the scent have endured.

The elegantly tooled label remains unchanged. The cologne is housed in a handsome gold-colored bottle, embellished with turquoise lettering.

Introduced	*1792*
Price	*Mid-range*

FRACAS

Scent Type
Floral
Composition
   Top Notes: *Bergamot, peach, orange blossom, greens*
   Heart Notes: *Tuberose, rose, jasmine, carnation, orris*
   Base Notes: *Sandalwood, cedarwood, moss, musk*

Famous Patrons
Beverly Sills

Fracas is a classic French floral bouquet, bursting with the white flowers for which Grasse is famous. Gentle fruits and fragrant woods round out the feminine floral scent, which was developed by Paris couturier Robert Piguet during World War II.

Piguet was known for his designs of simple elegance. During World War II, Nazi orders directed the top couture houses to relocate to Berlin. Piguet resisted and rode out the war in occupied Paris, continuing his work in fashion and fragrance. During this period he developed Fracas and Bandit, fragrant points of light in a dark time of history.

Look for Fracas in a black glass cube wrapped in pink tulle. Also available in bath products.

Introduced	*1945*
Price	*Mid-range*

FRED HAYMAN'S TOUCH

Scent Type
Floral
Composition
    Top Notes: *Living clementine, yellow rose, black violet*
    Heart Notes: *Wild lily of the valley, jonquil, purple carnation*
    Base Notes: *Exotic woods, peach, musk, vanilla*

Fred Hayman's Touch is an enchanting addition to the Fred Hayman family of fragrances. He describes the romantic floral scent as "soft enough to be worn during the day, yet spectacular enough for special evenings." It was created for the woman of adventure, intimacy and mystery.

The rectangular bottle is presented in an irresistibly touchable corduroy-like red box, embellished with the FH seal, gold-colored trim and sunny yellow border.

Look for it in fine department stores nationwide, or visit Fred Hayman's boutique at 273 North Rodeo Drive in Beverly Hills, where you can also enjoy *cappuccino* or Champagne at the bar, relax before the fireplace, shoot a game of pool, and select an elegant gown and accessories for the Academy Awards—all in one afternoon. It's what fabulous shopping should be. And while you're there, try his Personal Selections One and Six, scents that are available only at the Rodeo Drive store and a few select retailers.

As you may recall, Fred Hayman and former wife Gale Hayman established Giorgio, the Rodeo Drive store that spawned a best-selling fragrance as well as a best-selling novel—Judith Krantz's *Scruples*—and its sequel, *Scruples Two*. In 1993, Hayman's 273 boutique was once again in the limelight as a setting for the daytime television drama *Days of Our Lives*. For *Days* fans, Fred Hayman's was where characters Bo and Billie went on a wild shopping spree and were lavished with attention, not unlike regular customers at Hayman's establishment.

News Flash: At the time of writing, Hayman tells us he has plans for a new signature fragrance, called FJH or simply Freddy. We'll be on the lookout for another winner.

Introduced   1993
Price   *Mid-range*

GABRIELA SABATINI

Scent Type
Floral
Composition
    Top Notes: *Bergamot, lemon, greens*
    Heart Notes: *Tuberose, orange blossom, jasmine, lily of the valley, honeysuckle, heliotrope*
    Base Notes: *Vanilla, sandalwood, amber, moss*

In 1991, international tennis star Gabriela Sabatini introduced her signature fragrance from the Muelhens perfumery. The vivid floral bouquet is, in her words, "very sweet, very strong, very sensual, and very feminine." A scent as dynamic as Sabatini herself.

The black glass bottle is crowned with the GS logo, fashioned after a tennis ball. The line is packaged in hues of brilliant amethyst and gold.

Introduced   1991
Price   High range

GALANOS

Scent Type
    Floral - Oriental
Composition
    Top Notes: *Lily of the valley, gardenia*
    Heart Notes: *Red rose, jasmine, carnation, geranium*
    Base Notes: *Vanilla, cedarwood, oakmoss, tonka bean, musk, coriander, bay, clove, cypress*

Famous Patrons
    Nancy Reagan

From American-born James Galanos comes a well-bred signature fragrance. Galanos is known for his couture designs that grace women such as Nancy Reagan, Rosalind Russell and Diana Ross.

The genteel floral blend is amplified by Oriental background notes, exotic woods and fragrant spices that linger sensually on the skin. The feminine fragrance is housed in an elegant clear bottle of multiple curves and hollows.

Introduced   1979
Price   Mid-range

GALORE

Scent Type
    Floral - Oriental
Composition
    Top Notes: *Citrus, lily of the valley, ylang-ylang, narcissus*
    Heart Notes: *Carnation, jasmine, rose*
    Base Notes: *Amber, woods, musk*

French cosmetics entrepreneur Germaine Monteil submits Galore, a classic floral Oriental. Galore is amply endowed with French florals and warmed with woods, amber and long-lasting musk. A dusky, enchanting aroma.

Introduced   1964
Price   Mid-range

GARDENIA

Scent Type
    Floral
Composition
    Top Notes: *Absolutes of jasmine, orange blossom, tuberose*
    Heart Notes: *Clove, sage, pimiento*
    Base Notes: *Musk, patchouli, sandalwood, vetiver*

Coco Chanel's twenties version of Gardenia is a polished floral blend enhanced by a spicy accord and supported by sweet, powdery wooded notes. Gardenia bursts with the unforgettable essence of the finest French garden.

Perfect for tea in a spring garden, or a two-Evian power lunch. We imagine Chanel slipped Gardenia in her suitcase for her frequent French Riviera vacations.

Introduced   *1925*
Reintroduced   *1993*
Price   *Mid-range*

GARDÉNIA PASSION

Scent Type
    Single Floral
Composition
    Notes: *Gardenia*

Talented French perfumer Annick Goutal brings us Gardénia Passion. The scent is a heady harmony of pure gardenia. An intense, dramatic, unforgettable composition that is beautiful for afternoon tea, garden parties, walks in the park...or any place you want to sprinkle a little sunshine.

Annick Goutal has a knack for selecting and designing glamorous packaging. At Neiman Marcus we spotted a fabulous limited edition Louis XVI Baccarat flacon, filled with Gardénia Passion or Eau d'Hadrien. The bottle was hand decorated with delicate gold-colored flowers, topped with an old-fashioned atomizer spray, and beautifully presented in a velvet jewelry box with gold-colored cord accents.

Along with a variety of fragrance strengths, Gardénia Passion is also available in a sumptuous array of body and bath products.

Introduced   *1990*
Price   *Top range*

GEM

Scent Type
    Chypre - Fruity
Composition
    Top Notes: *Peach, plum, myrtle, cypress, cardamom, coriander, rosewood*
    Heart Notes: *Tuberose, jasmine, rose, clove, iris, ylang-ylang, carnation, orris*
    Base Notes: *Patchouli, vanilla, moss, amber, civet, vetiver*

Famous Patrons
    Actress Josette Banzet

The second fragrance offering from Van Cleef & Arpels, Gem is a rich chypre melange of rare floral essences, fresh fruits and exotic spices. Succulent fruits and spices create a distinctive top-drawer top note that gives way to a rich floral heart enhanced by spicy clove and carnation. Lingering base notes of sweet vanilla, patchouli and amber complete the feminine, dramatic fragrance.

Wish all of our gems came from Van Cleef & Arpels. Ahh...if only it were so....

Introduced   *1988*
Price   *High range*

GENNY SHINE

Scent Type
  Floral - Fruity
Composition
  Top Notes: *Freesia, aldehydes*
  Heart Notes: *Peach, apricot, rose, violet, iris, heliotrope, sandalwood*
  Base Notes: *Musk, vanilla, ambergris*

Genny Shine is a fragrance from Diana de Silva Cosmetiques, created in tandem with the Genny Oro evening wear collection.

Genny Shine is a radiant, invigorating fruity floral bouquet. Essence of peach, apricot and freesia impart a smooth sweetness, like biting into a juicy fresh-picked peach. Floral notes are blended with sandalwood and vanilla to extend the warm sweetness into the drydown phase. A fragrance of easy-wearing elegance, for career or fun, a perfect "let's do lunch" scent.

The fragrance is packaged in triangular glass Art Deco-inspired flacons, washed in delicate shades of peach and gold. It made its debut through its North American distributor, Gary Farn Ltd., at Bloomingdale's, Neiman Marcus and I. Magnin. Nothing like starting at the top.

Introduced   1993
Price   Mid-range

GIANFRANCO FERRE

Scent Type
  Floral

Composition
  Top Notes: *Hyacinth, bergamot, fruits, greens, coriander, orange blossom*
  Heart Notes: *Tuberose, jasmine, rose, honeysuckle, narcissus, lily of the valley, orchid*
  Base Notes: *Musk, spices, moss*

This is the first fragrance for women from the Italian fashion designer and architect, Gianfranco Ferre.

The sprightly floral bouquet is lifted by green herbal notes and warmed with musk, spices and moss. An easy-to-wear floral fragrance, it has an effect that is quiet and mannered, like a mountain-top stroll through the fragrant Italian gardens of Villa d'Este.

Introduced   1984
Price   Mid-range

GIORGIO BEVERLY HILLS

Scent Type
  Floral

Composition
  Top Notes: *Bergamot, mandarin, galbanum, greens, fruits*
  Heart Notes: *Jasmine, rose, carnation, ylang-ylang, orris, lily of the valley, hyacinth*
  Base Notes: *Sandalwood, cedarwood, musk, moss, amber*

Famous Patrons
   Nancy Reagan
   Farrah Fawcett
   Jacqueline Bisset
   Grace (Mrs. Harold) Robbins
   Former Vogue model Aly Spencer

Gale and Fred Hayman found immediate success with Giorgio, named after their internationally famous boutique on Rodeo Drive in the heart of Beverly Hills. The heady, exotic floral fragrance is a glamorous long-lasting scent. One of the best-selling fragrances of all times, it is dramatic and lavish, saucy and full of sexy verve...a fragrance to impress.

Giorgio set the stage for blockbuster fragrance hits of the eighties and nineties. The distinctive line, in its yellow and white striped packages, was unveiled at a million-dollar party. It was originally available only at the Rodeo Drive boutique and through mail order. Now, this bestseller can be found virtually worldwide. It is often copied, but never duplicated.

After years of hard work, entrepreneurs Gale and Fred Hayman sold the Giorgio Beverly Hills company to Avon for a handsome profit when they divorced in the eighties. Now Avon is enjoying the magic of Giorgio, along with two newer sibling fragrances, Red and Wings.

(Giorgio is a federally registered trademark of Giorgio Beverly Hills, Inc. ©1989 Fred Hayman Beverly Hills, Inc. and Giorgio Beverly Hills, Inc. are separate companies.)

Introduced	*1982*
Price	*Mid-range*

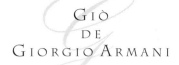

GIÒ
DE
GIORGIO ARMANI

Scent Type
   Floral - Fruity
Composition
   Top Notes: *Egyptian hyacinth, Sicilian mandarin*
   Heart Notes: *Green jasmine, tuberose, gardenia, red rose, ylang-ylang, clove, iris balm, peach, orange blossom*
   Base Notes: *Amber, sandalwood, vanilla*

Famous Patrons
   Model Lara Harris

Famed Italian designer Giorgio Armani created Giò to complement the timeless elegance and vivacity of his fashions. When you ask for it, pronounce it "Joe," as do those who know, for Giò is the diminutive form of Giorgio.

Armani is known for his understated approach to elegance, a spare simplicity that exudes glamour, reflected in his unconstructed silhouettes designed to drape the body. His fragrance imparts the same easy style. The rich, feminine floral begins with fruity top notes and the aroma of fresh flowers in bloom—achieved by new "living flower" technology that enables the perfumer to precisely reproduce the living scent, rather than the dried, distilled scent. Vivid notes of rose, gardenia and tuberose are balanced by spicy clove and spirited green jasmine, then tempered by warm base notes, making Giò as comfortable to wear as any Armani design.

Even the packaging is pure Armani—the rounded shoulders of the flacon are reminiscent of those on his classic unconstructed jackets. The only adornments are a weighted metal cap dipped in 24-karat gold and the gold leaf neck. And the inscription on the bottle? It is Armani's own signature, Giò.

Introduced   1993
Price   Top range

GIVENCHY III

Scent Type
  Chypre - Floral Animalic
Composition
  Top Notes: *Aldehydes, galbanum, peach, bergamot, gardenia*
  Heart Notes: *Jasmine, jonquil, carnation, rose, lily of the valley, orris*
  Base Notes: *Amber, patchouli, oakmoss, myrrh, vetiver, castoreum*

A harmonious classic from French couturier Hubert de Givenchy, this is a warm and natural woody floral scent. The contemporary chypre blend is available in a perfume and eau de toilette.

Introduced   1970
Price   Mid-range

GOLCONDA

Scent Type
  Floral
Composition
  Notes: *Floral essences*

An exotic floral fragrance whose name reaches back into history, Golconda is truly "an American in Paris." Although available in fine stores in North America, it hails from the elite Paris shop, Jars on Place Vendôme, a rare gem of a store owned by American jeweler Joel Rosenthal.

Rosenthal christened his scent Golconda after the ancient Indian province whose supply of the world's finest pink diamonds was depleted at the end of the seventeenth century. But don't forget your wallet—Golconda costs about $450 an ounce. Of course, that includes the Baccarat crystal bottle, a design inspired by a Golconda diamond belonging to Shah Jahan, an Indian ruler. The exotic letters carved in the Baccarat are similar to characters carved into the Shah's diamond. The stopper is a copy of a rough pink Golconda diamond.

You'll find this work of art crated and cushioned in dried Indian roses as though it had just made the ocean voyage in the bowels of a tall-masted ship, swept through time by the trade winds of our imagination. Perfect for your next voyage.

Introduced   1988
Price   Top range

GUCCI NO. 1

Scent Type
Floral - Aldehyde

Composition
Top Notes: Bergamot, aldehydes, lemon, hyacinth, rosewood, greens
Heart Notes: Rose carnation, jasmine, lilac, lily of the valley, heliotrope, orchid
Base Notes: Sandalwood, cedarwood, vanilla, amber, tonka bean, musk, vetiver

From the inimitable Gucci comes a Mediterranean floral bouquet, wrapped in Gucci red and green. Sparkling aldehydes create a breezy original top note. Soft florals and powdery woods complete the buoyant composition. And the eau de parfum is well-priced as compared to Gucci No. 3, a later introduction.

Introduced   1974
Price   Mid-range

GUCCI NO. 3

Scent Type
Chypre - Floral

Composition
Top Notes: Aldehydes, bergamot, coriander, calyx, greens
Heart Notes: Rose, jasmine, narcissus, tuberose, lily of the valley, orris
Base Notes: Amber, vetiver, patchouli, musk, moss, leather

Gucci No. 3 is a rich, radiant composition. The company says Gucci No. 3 is "a complex blend of stylish subtle influences that bespeak a distinctive European heritage. Warm, inviting ...worldly, sophisticated. Born of a tradition of impeccable taste and dedication to quality."

An Art Deco-inspired bottle sports frosted curved shoulders, a matching frosted stopper and a collar of Gucci red and green stripes. With exacting attention to detail, it's Gucci from head to toe.

Introduced   1985
Price   High range

GUESS?

Scent Type
Oriental - Ambery

Composition
Top Notes: Mandarin orange, grapefruit, lemon, black currant bud
Heart Notes: Orange blossom, jasmine, lily of the valley, hyacinth
Base Notes: Amber, oakmoss, patchouli, orris, sandalwood, vanilla

Famous Patrons
Model Claudia Schiffer
Drew Barrymore
Anna Nicole Smith

A youthful, invigorating scent from top sportswear designer Georges Marciano for Revlon. Guess? is a contemporary scent that opens with sassy fruits. Tempered by florals, it gives way to warm woods that leave an innocent aura of smoldering sexuality. In keeping with this image, Guess? features alluring bombshells in its provocative advertisements.

The Guess? trademark triangle is twisted to form the high-tech, high-impact bottle. The fashion scheme is black and white with a dash of red.

For those in strictly Guess? territory....

Introduced   1990
Price   High range

HABANITA

Scent Type
   Oriental - Ambery
Composition
   Top Notes: Bergamot, peach, orange blossom, raspberry
   Heart Notes: Rose, jasmine, ylang-ylang, orris, heliotrope, lilac
   Base Notes: Amber, oakmoss, leather, vanilla, musk, cedarwood, benzoin

Habanita is a warm Oriental blend from the Paris House of Molinard. Fruity top notes introduce the composition, which proceeds through rich florals to a final balsamic drydown of amber, leather, vanilla and musk. Sweet and sensual, beautiful for evening and cool crisp days.

The original Molinard was established in Grasse in 1849 to supply wealthy vacationers and royalty, including Queen Victoria. A Paris

presence was later established. The Grasse factory is now open for tours at certain times of the year. (60 blvd Victor-Hugo, telephone 93-36-01-62) Call ahead to the tourist office; this is a real treat!

Introduced   1921
Price   High range

HALSTON

Scent Type
   Chypre - Floral
Composition
   Top Notes: Melon, greens, peach, bergamot, spearmint, tagetes
   Heart Notes: Jasmine, rose, marigold, cedarwood, carnation, orris, ylang-ylang
   Base Notes: Vetiver, amber, patchouli, musk, sandalwood, incense, moss

The signature fragrance from Halston is a distinctive fragrance that has been a bestseller for years. The chypre blend opens with energizing green notes supported by smooth fruity essences, followed by a classic French floral bouquet that rests on an amber base. Easy to wear, easy to enjoy in a variety of bath and body products.

Introduced   1975
Price   High range

HEURE EXQUISE

Scent Type
 Floral
Composition
 Top and Heart Notes: *Florentine iris,*
 Turkish rose
 Base Notes: *Sandalwood*

Heure Exquise, which translates as "exquisite hour," is a romantically delicate scent. The refined essence of rose is combined with fragrant sandalwood. Creator Annick Goutal describes it as a fragrance for the "sublimely feminine woman."

Introduced   1986
Price   Top range

HISTOIRE D'AMOUR

Scent Type
 Chypre - Floral
Composition
 Top Notes: *Mandarin, bergamot,*
 basil, osmanthus
 Heart Notes: *Jasmine, rose, narcissus,*
 orange blossom, ylang-ylang, galbanum
 Base Notes: *Oakmoss, musk, patchouli*

In French, Histoire D'Amour means "love story." This scent from Parfums Aubusson is a chypre blend enhanced with rich florals and amber. The citrus top notes impart a significant lift to the composition.

Dedicated to love and femininity, the fragrance is bottled in a flacon engraved with cascading flowers, topped with a stopper in the shape of a fragile flower.

Introduced   1984
Price   Mid-range

HOT

Scent Type
 Oriental
Composition
 Top Notes: *Bergamot, rose, jasmine,*
 lily of the valley
 Heart Notes: *Spices, sandalwood,*
 cinnamon, bay leaf
 Base Notes: *Vanilla, amber, musk*

Hot is part of the Bill Blass trio of fragrances that includes Nude and Basic Black. A vivid Oriental composition, Hot has a spicy personality. The fragrance unfolds with rich florals and a tang of bergamot, quickly followed by exotic spices, sweet amber and long-lasting musk.

Hot is packaged in the hottest red to sizzle the senses. A wear-all-day, wear-all-night fragrance.

Introduced   1990
Price   High range

ICE WATER
BY
PINO SILVESTRE

Scent Type
   Floral
Composition
   Top Notes: *Bergamot, orange oil, lemon oil,*
   mandarin oil, clary sage, juniper berry, clove,
   lavender, thyme
   Heart Notes: *Lily of the valley, rose, jasmine,*
   geranium
   Base Notes: *Sandalwood, oakmoss,*
   cedarwood, amber, musk

From Europe comes a crisp floral fragrance
by Pino Silvestre. The initial splash of Ice
Water bursts with fresh citrus and spice notes.
The heart of the fragrance is a fountain of
extravagant flower essences, followed by base
notes of woods, musk and moss.

Introduced   *1993 (United States)*
Price   *Mid-range*

IL BACIO

Scent Type
   Floral - Fruity
Composition
   Top Notes: *Honeysuckle, rose, jasmine,*
   freesia, orchid, lily of the valley
   Heart Notes: *Peach, plum, melon,*
   passion fruit, pear, osmanthus, iris
   Base Notes: *Amber, sandalwood, violet,*
   musk, cedarwood

An understated fruity floral melange from
the Italian Princess Marcella di Borghese. Il

Bacio, Italian for "the kiss," is an airy, feminine
composition, created as a token of love. Il Bacio
features floral top notes, animated by a well-
rounded basket of succulent Mediterranean
fruits. A pretty springtime or light winter
fragrance, easy to wear for daytime.

Il Bacio is encased in a fan-shaped bottle
designed by Marc Rosen that the company says
is "reminiscent of the palazzo arches seen in
Venice." It is adorned by a knotted red cap,
suggesting the "unbreakable bond of eternal love."

Look for a Borghese lipstick in Il Bacio
Red, said to be the perfect kissing lipstick.
Venus would approve.

Introduced   *1993*
Price   *High range*

INFINI

Scent Type
   Floral - Aldehyde
Composition
   Top Notes: *Aldehydes, peach, bergamot,*
   neroli, coriander
   Heart Notes: *Rose, jasmine, lily of the valley,*
   carnation, ylang-ylang, orris
   Base Notes: *Sandalwood, musk, vetiver,*
   civet, tonka bean

From the House of Caron comes Infini,
a floral with scintillating aldehydic top notes.
The feminine bouquet is nestled in soft wooded
background notes. Its subtle, ethereal quality is
fitting for casual or professional daytime wear.

The bottle was conceived by Serge Mansau, a respected bottle designer. The clear glass flacon has a diamond-shaped cutout in the heart, matched by another diamond cutout in the angular crystal stopper. Crisp, asymmetrical lines complete the attractive object of art.

Introduced   1970
Price   High range

ISIS

Scent Type
Floral
Composition
  Top Notes: *White rose*
  Heart and Base Notes: *White violet, bird of paradise*

Famous Patrons
  Princess Diana of Wales

William Owen calls the delicate Isis "a perfume that stimulates the imagination, awakens the senses to the beauty and mystery of romance that lies within our reach." He developed Isis as a challenge to re-create the fleeting essence of white rose and violet. As with Owen's fragrance Adoration, Isis was produced for Princess Diana. The natural fragrance is derived from the type of flowers grown at William Owen's estate on the coast of Wales.

All Wm. Owen brand fragrances are designed to be worn alone, or layered and mixed with others in the collection. Owen encourages experimentation and often refers to his scents as "moods." Isis is a light thoroughbred blend of romantic flowers, quite feminine. Beautiful for daytime, glamorous for evening.

Isis was the Egyptian goddess of fertility, wife of Osiris, god of regeneration. Naturally, Owen also offers the fragrance Osiris for men.

Isis is available in cologne and perfume, in plain or jewel-encrusted flacons. The signature stone for this fragrance is "Swarovski golden topaz," set amidst brilliant Austrian crystals in 22-karat gold. William Owen was kind enough to send us our very own Isis to try, in a gold-colored moire box tucked inside an elaborate outer box of champagne silk brocade. The French cut crystal flacon was wrapped with a delicate gold-colored cord. A magnificent presentation from a talented man with a exquisite eye for detail.

Introduced   1988
Price   Mid- to High range

IVOIRE

Scent Type
Floral - Green

Composition

Top Notes: Jasmine, galbanum, bergamot, violet, mandarin, aldehydes
Heart Notes: Turkish rose, lily of the valley, Tuscany ylang-ylang, carnation, pepper, nutmeg, cinnamon, berry pepper
Base Notes: Vetiver, oakmoss, sandalwood, labdanum, amber, vanilla, patchouli, tonka bean

From couturier Pierre Balmain, Ivoire is a green floral aroma, voluptuous and seductive, yet in an offhand, innocent manner. The name was supposedly inspired by a woman at a gala who was dressed in creamy pale silk, stark among a sea of black tuxedos.

The sophisticated floral unravels with shimmering green top notes, flowing into a floral heart accented with spices and greens. The long-lasting base is composed of sweet amber and powdery woods.

After working with many fashion legends—Christian Dior, Lucien Lelong, Robert Piguet and Edward Molyneux—Pierre Balmain opened his boutique in Paris in 1946, where his designs were sought after by a privileged clientele. Before his death in 1982, he was honored as an Officer of the Legion of Honor, one of France's most esteemed positions.

Look for Ivoire products in creme and gold-colored packaging, as though dressed for a ball like the mysterious woman in pale silk.

Introduced	*1979*
Price	*High range*

JARDINS DE BAGATELLE

Scent Type
Floral

Composition

Top Notes: Violet, aldehydes, lemon, bergamot
Heart Notes: Orange blossom, tuberose, magnolia, gardenia, rose, jasmine, ylang-ylang, orchid, lily of the valley, narcissus
Base Notes: Cedarwood, vetiver, patchouli, musk

A classic floral garden fragrance from Jean-Paul Guerlain, Jardins de Bagatelle was created for the modern woman. Like most Guerlain fragrances, it carries with it an enchanting tale. It was inspired by and named after Queen Marie Antoinette's gardens and château in the Bois de Boulogne, built for her in 1777. As in her gardens, spring florals blossom into a full-bodied white floral heart. The magic of white flowers is fragrant, long-lasting sweetness. Jardins de Bagatelle is a versatile, feminine fragrance that blooms from sunrise to sunset.

The romantic Bagatelle retreat was the result of a wager. Legend has it that one day the Queen and the Count of Artois, who was brother to Louis XVI, were enjoying a horseback ride through the French countryside. When they came upon a decrepit chalet, the Count bet the Queen that he would build a new château for amusement on the site in less than ten weeks. She took the bet, and in less than sixty-four days, Bagatelle was built. Though she lost the bet, she loved the new château and gardens.

As with most Guerlain fragrances, the scent was conceived as a reflection of its time. Jardins de Bagatelle was designed in the eighties for the woman who is joyful and assertive, yet still feminine at heart.

Jardins de Bagatelle is available in an eau de toilette, as well as bath and body care products.

Introduced   1983
Price   Mid-range

JE REVIENS

Scent Type
Floral - Aldehyde
Composition
Top Notes: *Orange blossom, aldehydes, bergamot, violet*
Heart Notes: *Clove, rose, jasmine, hyacinth, lilac, orris, ylang-ylang*
Base Notes: *Amber, incense, tonka bean, vetiver, musk, moss, sandalwood*

The couture House of Worth brings forth Je Reviens, a popular scent for more than sixty years. The fragrance opens with bright aldehydic top notes, then meanders along a floral path liberally doused with rare spices. Smoky incense and mellow amber linger long after the company has gone home.

Englishman Charles Frederick Worth established his fashion salon in Paris 1858, catering to a clientele of wealth and royalty, including the Empress Eugénie. From his shop on the chic rue de la Paix, he saw clients by personal referral only. Flowing, fluid garments became his trademark. His sons, Jean-Philippe and Gaston Worth, continued the business and created fragrances to give to clients, scents that proved so popular they were soon sold on a wider scale, an endeavor managed by great-grandson Roger Worth.

Je Reviens means "I will return." And it does, again and again. A perennial favorite. Look for Je Reviens in the blue aquamarine boxes.

Introduced   1932
Price   Mid-range

JEAN-PAUL GAULTIER

Scent Type
Floral - Fruity
Composition
Top Notes: *Bulgarian rose, Chinese star anise, Tunisian orange blossom, Italian tangerine*
Heart Notes: *Indian ginger, orchid, Florentine iris, ylang-ylang, rose, orange blossom*
Base Notes: *Réunion Island vanilla, amber, musk*

Famous Patrons
Madonna

Flamboyant French designer Jean-Paul Gaultier offers a fragrance that's sure to raise a few eyebrows. Gaultier catapulted to international fame after Madonna displayed his conical corsets and fashions during her 1991 *Blond Ambition* tour.

The signature fragrance is a fruity floral, with a top note reminiscent of scented nail polish and face powder, scents that Gaultier remembered from childhood and wanted to reproduce.

The packaging is equally outrageous; the glass is molded into the shape of a corseted bust. The flacon was inspired by an earlier "torso" perfume bottle from Roman designer Elsa Schiaparelli, whose 1937 hyacinth and patchouli perfume was called Shocking. It was sold in a bottle modeled after a Venus de Milo bust that she received from her friend Mae West.

The Jean-Paul Gaultier perfume is further adorned by a metal corset, while a soft drink tab forms the stopper. Look for it in the tin can package. Pure Gaultier, pure avant-garde.

Introduced   1993
Price   High range

JESSICA MCCLINTOCK

Scent Type
    Floral - Green
Composition
    Top Notes: *Black currant bud, bergamot, basil, ylang-ylang*
    Heart Notes: *Rose, white jasmine, lily of the valley*
    Base Notes: *Musk, woods*

American designer Jessica McClintock is known for her delicate, flowing fantasy creations. To complement her designs, she created her signature fragrance, a scent as romantic and feminine as her fashions.

The fragrance owes its fruity green top notes to bergamot and basil, with a touch of cassis, the black currant fruit. The heart is a delicate, sparkling blend of classic florals, bolstered by musky background notes. The potion is packaged in clear glass bottles with lacy white and silver accents.

A sweet scent for daytime and soft evening wear; ideal for the incurable romantic in all of us.

Introduced   1989
Price   Mid-range

JICKY

Scent Type
    Fougère
Composition
    Top Notes: *Bergamot, lemon, mandarin*
    Heart Notes: *Lavender, rosemary, basil, orris, tonka bean*
    Base Notes: *Vanilla, amber, benzoin, rosewood, spices, leather*

Jicky is a fresh fougère from Guerlain that has endured for more than a century. Citrus, lavender, vanilla and amber form the dominant accords of the classic fragrance, a scent that is shared by men and women.

The Jicky story began in the 1850s when Aimé Guerlain was living in England, studying chemistry and medicine. He fell in love with a woman he nicknamed Jicky. All was bliss until his aging father, Pierre François Pascal, summoned him back to Paris to take over the family business. When he asked for Jicky's hand in marriage, her family would not allow it. So he returned to Paris alone and brokenhearted.

More than thirty years later, Aimé Guerlain honored the great love of his life by creating a fragrance that bore her nickname. He was proud of the breakthrough modern blend that utilized revolutionary technology in the perfumer's palette.

For the floral notes, he discovered a new solvent technology that produced a potent pure flower essence. For the base accord, he employed another of his discoveries, synthesis, which came from a gum resin called benzoin. From this he extracted vanillin, a substance that shared the dominant theme of natural vanilla but lacked the background complexities. Guerlain found that when he blended vanilla and vanillin for the base note of Jicky, the result was a rounder, full-bodied scent. Jicky was a new breed of fragrance.

But the year was 1889, and respectable women wore light, single flower scents such as lavender, violet or rose, or simple bouquets. With its notes of citrus, florals, woods and spices, Jicky was considered strong and scandalous among proper ladies. The only women who wore such distinctive fragrances were prostitutes, who presumably mixed fragrances so potential clients could identify them on the dark streets.

Indeed, men appreciated Jicky. Soon men who wanted to be slightly provocative began to wear it. By 1912 women's fashion magazines began to praise it and women embraced the complex fragrance once considered scandalous. Today, more than one hundred years later, the original formula Jicky remains popular with women and men, and Aimé Guerlain's great love has become a legend.

Introduced   1889
Price   High range

JIL SANDER No. 4

Scent Type
  Floral - Oriental
Composition
  Top Notes: *Light rose, geranium, peach, plum, galbanum*
  Heart Notes: *Violets, jasmine, rose, tuberose, heliotrope, ylang-ylang, carnation, tarragon, myrrh*
  Base Notes: *Grey ambergris, moss, sandalwood, patchouli, vanilla, musk*

Famous Patrons
  Kim Bassinger
  Jacqueline Kennedy Onassis

Jil Sander is a German-born fashion design purist. Her No. 4 fragrance is introduced with a green fruity top note, followed by a delicate flowery heart enhanced with dry spices. The subtle Oriental background trails a sensual mix of woods, ambergris and vanilla. Modern, minimalist, a spare yet opulent fragrance. Her scent is the personification of today's woman—independent, successful, charismatic. No. 4 is inherently seductive, like the Jil Sander fashions that have garnered international acclaim and industry awards.

The fragrance is housed in a clear cylinder accented with hues of black and gold. Bath and body products are also available. For purity of style, experience Jil Sander creations.

Introduced   1992
Price   High range

JOLIE MADAME

Scent Type
   Chypre - Floral Animalic
Composition
   Top Notes: *Gardenia, artemisia, bergamot, coriander, neroli*
   Heart Notes: *Jasmine, tuberose, rose, jonquil, orris*
   Base Notes: *Patchouli, oakmoss, vetiver, musk, castoreum, leather, civet*

Jolie Madame is a happy fragrance from Pierre Balmain. Always ladylike, the dry chypre opens with sprightly top notes, followed by a dry floral heart. A warm mossy background completes the well-mannered composition.

For more information on the fascinating life of Pierre Balmain, read his 1964 autobiography, *My Years and Seasons*.

Introduced   1953
Price   High range

JOOP! POUR FEMME

Scent Type
   Floral - Oriental
Composition
   Top Notes: *Neroli, bergamot*
   Heart Notes: *Bulgarian rose, jasmine, orange blossom*
   Base Notes: *Vanilla, sandalwood, patchouli, coumarin*

From Parfums Joop!, German designer Wolfgang Joop introduces his version of a floral Oriental, distributed by Lancaster Group in North America. Pronounce it "yope," to rhyme with "hope."

Beginning with a fresh citrus top note, Joop! dissolves into a rich heart note, then gives way to a sensual symphony of warm, exotic Oriental essences. Bursting with Joop! impact. Great for the trendy young "let's do lunch" bunch.

Introduced   1991
Price   Top range

JOY

Scent Type
Floral

Composition

Top Notes: Aldehydes, peach, greens, calyx
Heart Notes: Jasmine, Bulgarian rose,
ylang-ylang, orchid, lily of the valley,
orris, tuberose
Base Notes: Sandalwood, musk, civet

Famous Patrons

Mary Pickford
Gloria Swanson
Woolworth heiress Barbara Hutton
Actress Constance Bennett
Patou assistant, social journalist Elsa Maxwell

In 1930, the legendary Joy was introduced as the costliest perfume in the world. French couturier Jean Patou had set out to create a fragrance "free from all vulgarity" at any cost, as well as "impudent, crazy and extravagant beyond reason." Indeed, the sumptuous scent quickly became revered as the world's most extravagant perfume and to this day remains the costliest perfume to produce, according to the Patou firm.

The dominant notes are absolute of jasmine and Bulgarian rose, two of the world's rarest and most expensive essences. Each ounce contains the essence from more than 10,000 jasmine flowers and twenty-eight dozen roses. Lavish quantities of the delicate jasmine and elegant rose are woven into a rich tapestry of more than a hundred essences, resulting in a scent that remains true to Jean Patou's vision. Each vessel of fragrance is still mixed and hand-sealed as it was at its inception in a process carefully overseen by Jean Kerléo, Patou's internationally recognized in-house perfumer, along with Patou's great nephews, who head the company.

Jean Patou launched his quest for Joy in 1926 when he took his assistant, cafe society woman Elsa Maxwell, with him to Grasse to work with perfumers on the new scent. Together they searched for a fragrance that would meet the exacting requirements of the best-dressed and most discriminating women of the world, the social leaders and accomplished women of their day. After exhaustive testing they were were presented with the formula for Joy, a recipe that called for twice the amount of essential oils that other popular perfumes contained. But alas, the perfumer told them it was too expensive to be commercially viable. That cinched it. Hence was born the "costliest fragrance in the world," and women the world over had to have it.

Joy is timeless; as revered today as it was more than sixty years ago. It remains a strong, dynamic floral essence with an unmistakable stamp of wealth, breeding and confidence. For a special treat, indulge in Joy in Baccarat crystal, one perfect ounce of pure joy for about $585—and worth every penny.

Introduced   1930
Price   *Top range*

K DE KRIZIA

Scent Type
   Floral

Composition
   Top Notes: Aldehydes, peach, hyacinth,
   bergamot, neroli
   Heart Notes: Jasmine, narcissus,
   orange blossom, rose, carnation, orchid,
   lily of the valley, orris
   Base Notes: Sandalwood, vetiver, musk,
   amber, moss, civet, vanilla, styrax, leather

K de Krizia hails from the House of Krizia,
purveyor of fine fashions, fragrance, resorts and
more. Slip into K with a spritz of fresh aldehydes. Sophisticated florals weave through the
heart, leading to a warm woody base laced with
soft leather and vanilla. A versatile day-to-
evening fragrance.

Introduced	1981
Price	High range

KENZO

Scent Type
   Floral

Composition
   Top Notes: Mandarin, orange blossom,
   bergamot, greens, spices
   Heart Notes: Tuberose, jasmine, rose,
   lily of the valley, carnation, orris, coriander,
   cumin, cedarwood, sandalwood
   Base Notes: Amber, vetiver, musk,
   moss, patchouli

Japanese fashion designer Kenzo interprets
the floral bouquet with his namesake fragrance.
Kenzo blossoms with a full floral heart, lightened by crisp top notes of fruits and greens.
Sweet amber mingles with woods and musk
to cast a lingering spell.

The floral concoction comes in a rounded
flacon of frosted glass, crowned with an intricate
carved flower. Pure Kenzo style.

Introduced	1988
Price	High range

KL

Scent Type
   Oriental - Spicy

Composition
   Top Notes: Orange, bergamot, spices
   Heart Notes: Clove, cinnamon, pimento,
   rose, jasmine, ylang-ylang, orchid
   Base Notes: Amber, myrrh, vanilla,
   patchouli, labdanum, olibanum,
   benzoin, civet, styrax

From designer Karl Lagerfeld and Parfums International comes an enduring scent, Lagerfeld's signature KL. A spicy Oriental fragrance, it also sports fruity top notes that dissolve into smoldering florals steeped in warm ambery balsamics. The result is a soft Oriental that glides through the seasons; an imminently wearable fragrance from a master designer.

Karl Lagerfeld is a contemporary couturier, born in Hamburg, Germany, in 1939. He entered the world of Parisian haute couture while still a teenager, and designed for top fashion houses such as Patou, Balmain, Chloé, Fendi and Chanel, as well as his own line, Lagerfeld. A recognized trend-setter, he imprints his style on women's and men's collections, even popularizing his own sleek ponytail hairstyle for men, a hot haute look.

The bottle is a Marc Rosen design, reminiscent of an arched fan in shades of amber, gold and pearl gray. Lagerfeld is often seen carrying a fan, one of his favorite accoutrements. He has a vast fan collection, and has donated many to museums.

KL is a fragrance of timeless sophistication, as reflected in Lagerfeld's collections for the House of Chanel.

Introduced	*1983*
Price	*High range*

KNOWING

Scent Type
Chypre - Floral

Composition
   Top Notes: *Greens, coriander, orange, aldehydes*
   Heart Notes: *Rose, jasmine, lily of the valley, cedarwood, cardamom*
   Base Notes: *Amber, sandalwood, patchouli, spices, vetiver, orris, oakmoss*

Knowing is an understated composition, redolent of fragrant woods and soft spring flowers with a final aura of oakmoss and spice. Another fine fragrance from Estée Lauder.

Introduced	*1988*
Price	*Top range*

L'AIR DU TEMPS

Scent Type
Floral
Composition
   Top Notes: *Bergamot, peach, rosewood, neroli*
   Heart Notes: *Gardenia, carnation, jasmine, May rose, ylang-ylang, orchid, lily, clove, orris*
   Base Notes: *Ambergris, musk, vetiver, benzoin, cedarwood, moss, sandalwood, spices*

L'Air du Temps is a classic French fragrance from the Parisian firm of Nina Ricci. The fragrance is like a bouquet of spring flowers strewn in the sun across a bed of precious woods and subtle spices. L'Air du Temps is an easy-to-wear floral scent that floats effortlessly from day to evening. Graceful, feminine, innocent and understated.

Italian-born Nina Ricci opened her couture boutique in 1932 amidst worldwide uncertainty. Closed in 1939 during World War II, the business reopened six years later under her son, Robert Ricci. Before her death in 1970, Nina Ricci was awarded the French Legion of Honor for her collections and accomplishments.

The lovely flacon was designed by Robert Ricci—a pair of doves swoon atop the stopper, wings spread, beaks touching—a timeless image of love. As it was in 1948, the perfume is sold in crystal Lalique flacons of various hues. Each year a limited edition is offered, signed and numbered. Beautiful for gifts or to spoil yourself.

Introduced   1948
Price   High range

L'ARTE DE GUCCI

Scent Type
  Chypre - Floral
Composition
  Top Notes: *Bergamot, fruits, coriander, aldehydes, greens*
  Heart Notes: *Rose, jasmine, lily of the valley, mimosa, tuberose, narcissus, geranium, orris*
  Base Notes: *Amber, musk, oakmoss, patchouli, leather, vetiver*

A rich fragrance composition from Gucci— the Art of Gucci. The chypre blend begins with citrus and fruits, followed by a rosy floral heart and a cozy wooded drydown. Available in eau de parfum and eau de toilette fragrance strengths.

Introduced   1991
Price   High range

L'HEURE BLEUE

Scent Type
  Floral - Ambery
Composition
  Top Notes: *Bergamot, lemon, coriander, neroli*
  Heart Notes: *Bulgarian rose, iris, heliotrope, jasmine, ylang-ylang, orchid*
  Base Notes: *Vanilla, sandalwood, musk, vetiver, benzoin*

Famous Patrons
  Catherine Deneuve
  Queen Elizabeth II

L'Heure Bleue means "blue hour" in French, and it was reportedly inspired by the gentle blue-hued twilight of a pre-World War I Paris, a time of relative innocence.

Third-generation perfumer Jacques Guerlain conceived the fragrance for sophisticated, romantic women of distinction. He freely employed the latest synthetic ingredients to create a totally new scent, combined with passionate florals and dusky, exotic base notes including vanilla, musk and aromatic woods. The resulting scent is tender yet penetrating, like a twilit evening in Paris, with undercurrents of bewitching sensuality.

L'Heure Bleue was a landmark scent of 1912 and remains an enchanting favorite.

The perfume is captured in a heavy glass flacon. Scrollwork adorns the shoulders. The triangular stopper is shaped like a gentleman's hat, a *chapeau de gendarme*, from which a hand-tied silken tassel dangles. An elegant presentation fitting of the fragrance itself.

Introduced   1912
Price   High range

L'INSOLENT

Scent Type
    Floral
Composition
    Top Notes: *Bergamot, mandarin, cassie, peach, pineapple*
    Heart Notes: *Tuberose, jasmine, orange blossom, lily of the valley, coriander, carnation, rosewood*
    Base Notes: *Amber, oakmoss, patchouli, musk, vanilla, cedarwood*

L'Insolent is one of a trio of women's fragrances from French high fashion designer Charles Jourdan. L'Insolent is unabashedly feminine, with fruity top notes, exotic florals and sweet vanilla smoothed into a sensual, woody Oriental base. Wear it when you want to be at your arrogant best.

Introduced   1986
Price   Mid-range

L'INTREDIT

Scent Type
    Floral - Aldehyde
Composition
    Top Notes: *Aldehydes, mandarin, peach, bergamot, strawberry*
    Heart Notes: *Jasmine, rose, jonquil, narcissus, lily of the valley, orris, ylang-ylang*
    Base Notes: *Sandalwood, vetiver, musk, amber, cistus, benzoin, tonka bean*

Famous Patrons
    Audrey Hepburn

Renowned French couturier Hubert Givenchy created this aldehydic floral bouquet for actress Audrey Hepburn. It is said that for many years, Hepburn was the only woman allowed to wear the feminine fragrance. Givenchy was one of her favorite designers and created many of her clothes for films such as *Breakfast at Tiffany's*.

L'Intredit is a smooth blend of elegant floral notes in perfect harmony with bright aldehydes and succulent fruits. Balsamic base notes create an understated sensual aura. If fragrance were a movie scene, L'Intredit would be the opening sequence of *Breakfast at Tiffany's* with Hepburn draped in a black Givenchy evening dress gazing into the Tiffany window of sparkling jewels. Quietly alluring, spare sophistication.

Introduced   1957
Price   High range

LA PRAIRIE

Scent Type
Floral - Fruity
Composition
Top Notes: *Bulgarian rose, honeysuckle, peach, tagetes, osmanthus, peony, violet leaves*
Heart Notes: *Orange blossom, peach, plum, tuberose, heliotrope, rose*
Base Notes: *Sandalwood, amber, oakmoss, patchouli, musk, cedarwood*

The signature fragrance from the esteemed Swiss cosmetic company is La Prairie, a bright, rich blend of succulent fruits, energetic greens and sweet floral notes.

Housed in a collection of cut crystal frosted flacons, and crowned in hues of platinum and blue, La Prairie will grace any fine lady's boudoir with quiet elegance. As the company says, it is "the fragrance for one woman in a thousand." Look for it at La Prairie counters.

Introduced   1993
Price   *High range*

LAGUNA

Scent Type
Floral - Fresh
Composition
Top Notes: *Moroccan lemon, Calabrian tangerine, Spanish verbena, Asian green galbanum, plum, pineapple*
Heart Notes: *Egyptian rose, Italian iris, lily of the valley, jasmine*
Base Notes: *Madagascar sandalwood, Réunion Island vanilla, amber, musk, coconut, cedarwood, patchouli*

A recent addition to the fragrance line of the late artist Salvador Dali is this shimmering fresh floral. Packed with exotic fruits and spicy iris, the modern eau de toilette was created for a youthful clientele. Refreshing, light and "slightly impertinent," Laguna is said to have drawn its inspiration from the Pacific Ocean. Indeed, the fragrance is ideal for warm summer days or a plunge in a clear lagoon.

The fragrance flows in the trademark Salvador Dali flacon—a frosted glass rendering of voluptuous lips with a nose-shaped stopper. Outrageously fun! The outer package is colored in pale Caribbean Sea turquoise and embellished with Dali's signature. A 1981 Dali painting, *Apparition of the Face of Aphrodite of Knidos in a Landscape*, served as inspiration for the unusual packaging.

Introduced   1991
Price   *Mid-range*

LALIQUE

Scent Type
Floral

Composition
Top Notes: Chinese gardenia,
Sicilian mandarin, blackberry
Heart Notes: Grasse magnolia,
Tunisian orange blossom, peony,
Bulgarian rose, ylang-ylang
Base Notes: Réunion Island vanilla,
Virginia cedarwood, East Indian sandalwood,
Tibetan musk, Colombian amber,
Yugoslavian oakmoss

Famous Patrons
Marie-Claude Lalique, designer of beautiful
crystal collectible artwork

Lalique is a namesake fragrance from Lalique, maker of fine collectible glassware. The founder of the company, René Lalique, first collaborated with François Coty in 1906 to elevate the art form of the perfume bottle. Today, granddaughter Marie-Claude Lalique brings her vision of perfume and flacons full circle with a fragrance inspired by her gardens in Provence.

From her fragrant flowering oasis spill forth blossoms of magnolia and peony, her favorites, and the main floral scents of the Lalique perfume. The challenge was to create these two essences by blending other essences from the perfumer's palette, for they do not exist as essential oils. This task accomplished, the blend was enlivened with touches of blackberry and mandarin, then softened with Colombian amber. Base notes of

musk, vanilla and woods create a long-lasting aura. The result is a subtle refined fragrance, remarkably like a Provençal spring garden.

The fragrance resides in a package of vivid turquoise and understated terra cotta, and is draped with a gift: A crystal pendant suspended from a silk cord that can be worn as a necklace. Inside rests a flacon of clear and satin-finished mouth-blown crystal. Frosted trellises of sculpted leaves embrace the transparent center vial. The leafy vine motif is continued on the stopper and the crystal pendant.

Each year, Marie-Claude Lalique creates a new bottle collection. For 1994 she designed "The Four Muses," an elongated bottle with a half-draped female form sculpted into each of four sides. Her special collections are available in a limited number of stores, including Neiman Marcus and select Bloomingdale's. Highly collectible.

Introduced	1992
Price	*Top range*

LAURA ASHLEY NO. 1

Scent Type
Floral - Fruity

Composition
Top Notes: Peach, hyacinth, bergamot,
gardenia, galbanum
Heart Notes: Narcissus, rose, jasmine,
orchid, clove, carnation
Base Notes: Sandalwood, musk,
vanilla, cyclamen

A soft floral fragrance is submitted by romantic designer Laura Ashley. No. 1 is a subtle, delicate scent that reverberates with the essence of white flowers.

It is said that this fragrance was presented as an anniversary gift to Laura Ashley from her husband. No. 1 is sweet and feminine, befitting the romance of Laura Ashley clothing and home designs.

The eau de parfum comes in glass flacons etched with red, yellow and green flowers, while the eau de toilette is in classic clear bottles; both are housed in ivory packaging. The fragrance is also available in an array of bath and body products.

Introduced	*1989*
Price	*High range*

LAUREN

Scent Type
   Floral - Fruity
Composition
   Top Notes: *Wild marigold, greens, rosewood, pineapple*
   Heart Notes: *Bulgarian rose, lilac, violet, jasmine, lily of the valley, cyclamen*
   Base Notes: *Cedarwood, oakmoss, sandalwood, vetiver, carnation*

From American designer Ralph Lauren hails a light contemporary, feminine floral fragrance. Lauren opens with energizing greens and fruits, followed by a floral harmony with delicate undertones of spices and woods. As natural as the elegantly tailored, easy-to-wear Ralph Lauren designs—all timeless American classics.

Ralph Lauren explains: "My philosophy about fragrance, like fashion, is simple: Never accept substitutes for the best. And if the best doesn't exist, create it."

The understated fragrance is presented in ruby red flacons, accented with gold-colored caps. The clear lead crystal perfume flacon was inspired by antique regency inkwells and is now part of the permanent collection of the Cooper-Hewitt Museum in New York.

The classic Lauren scent also comes is a wide array of bath and body products, many in plastic bottles with flip-tops; great for traveling. One of our favorites is the perfumed body creme, rich in softening emollients and enhanced by gold-colored sparkles that leave a glittering golden veil on the body. Beautiful on the skin when the sunlight kisses it—a must for summer shoulders.

Introduced	*1978*
Price	*High range*

LE DIX

Scent Type
   Floral - Aldehyde
Composition
   Top Notes: *Aldehydes, peach, lemon, bergamot, coriander*
   Heart Notes: *Jasmine, rose, orris, lilac, lily of the valley*
   Base Notes: *Vetiver, sandalwood, musk, amber, tonka bean, benzoin, Peru balsam*

Le Dix is a classic fragrance from the celebrated Spanish couturier Cristobal Balenciaga. Le Dix debuted in Paris in 1947, the same year Christian Dior introduced his New Look collection of post-World War II fashion. Le Dix was one of the new postwar fragrances eagerly sought out by women—and their men—who had denied themselves of luxuries for far too long during the war.

Balenciaga was born in northern Spain, but moved to Paris in 1937 during the Spanish Civil War. Creator of the pillbox hat, three-quarter sleeves and flamenco dresses, he also trained other young designers with names like Ungaro and Courrèges. He designed for women of wealth and title, including those of the Spanish royal family. Look for Balenciaga couture in the New York Metropolitan Museum collection.

Le Dix is French for "ten," named for his salon at No. 10, avenue Georges V, and indeed, it scores a perfect ten with us.

Introduced   1947
Price   High range

LES FLEURS DE CLAUDE MONET

Scent Type
Floral
Composition
Top Notes: Iris, lily of the valley
Heart Notes: Lavender, jasmine, daffodil, white roses
Base Notes: Ambergris

Imagine the floral aromas that Claude Monet may have breathed in as he painted his ethereal landscapes, brimming with flowers, bursting with color and light. Imagine that and you will capture the essence of the fragrance Les Fleurs de Claude Monet, an enchanting bouquet of the artist's favorite flowers, inspired by his pastoral paintings of the gardens at Giverny, his beloved French home.

Introduced   1991
Price   Mid-range

LÉONARD DE LÉONARD

Scent Type
Floral - Green
Composition
Top Notes: Iris aldehydes, galbanum, hyacinth, lemon, bergamot
Heart Notes: Rose, orris, lily of the valley, carnation, ylang-ylang
Base Notes: Musk, sandalwood, moss, amber, cedarwood, spices

From Léonard Parfums of Paris comes a green floral blend couched in a powdery wooded base. The dominant floral note is a slightly spicy iris aldehyde. Vivid, sparkling, breezy.

Léonard de Léonard is also available in bath and body products.

Introduced   1989
Price   Mid-range

LISTEN

Scent Type
    Floral - Fruity
Composition
    Top Notes: *Marigold, ylang-ylang,*
    lily of the valley, tangerine, bergamot
    Heart Notes: *Jasmine, rose, gardenia,*
    violet, lilac
    Base Notes: *Musk, vetiver*

Listen is a lyrical floral bouquet with a fresh fruit accent. Composed by jazz musician Herb Alpert, Listen is an olfactory translation of musical impulses, an effervescent orchestration.

Crisp notes of bergamot and tangerine set the stage for a feminine heart with notes of jasmine, rose, gardenia and other light florals. The bouquet is warmed with the aromatic wooded note of vetiver, while musk adds tenacity and a lingering sensuality. An easy-to-wear fragrance for day to evening.

Many perfumers say that they can actually see a fragrance, or in Alpert's case, hear the fragrance. This process is called synthesia, and is the sympathetic response of one sense to another, hence one may hear colors or see aromas. Synthesia enables a multifarious artist such as Alpert to draw on all senses in the artistic process.

Nineteenth-century art critic and theoretician Walter Pater once said, "All the arts aspire to the condition of music." Alpert's musical finesse aids him as a polyartist in applying his interpretive vision to different fields. The worlds of music and perfumery benefit, as does the world of painting, for Alpert is also a painter of distinction. No doubt his jazz style prompted him to emulate the Abstract Impressionists, with vivid color and fluid interpretations that garner worldwide recognition.

Listen's bottle and packaging also reflect the polyartistic synthesis. The flacon borrows its shape from the trumpet and was designed by renowned French bottle designer Pierre Dinand. Outer packaging sports vibrant tones of violet, burgundy and tangerine in fluid lines, similar to an Alpert jazz melody.

Introduced   1989
Price   *Mid-range*

LIU

Scent Type
    Floral - Aldehyde
Composition
    Top Notes: *Bergamot, neroli, aldehydes*
    Heart Notes: *Jasmine, May rose, iris*
    Base Notes: *Amber, vanilla, woods*

Every Guerlain fragrance begins with a story, before the first drop of essential oil is selected. The delicate Liu was inspired by a character from Puccini's opera *Turandot.*

Guerlain created Liu more than six decades ago, a charming romantic fragrance featuring a dominant bouquet of jasmine, rose and iris. Exhilarating citrus top notes and powdery base notes round out the floral aldehyde composition. Inspired by a woman of tenderness and passion whose love and generosity are boundless, Liu is understated, refined. A subtle fragrance, ideal for the professional woman with a multifaceted life.

Guerlain submitted this outline of *Turandot*:

In the opera, the Princess Turandot dares any prince or nobleman who seeks her hand in marriage to successfully answer three riddles or be sentenced to death.

One of her suitors, the Unknown Prince, accepts the challenge and proffers triumphant responses to the riddles, thereby winning the Princess's hand. Sensitive to the Princess's opposition to the marriage, however, the Prince offers Turandot a challenge of his own: If she can guess his name, he will relinquish his right to her hand.

The desperate princess kidnaps Timur, the Prince's father, and threatens to torture him until he reveals the guarded secret. To save Timur's life, Liu, the Prince's servant, acknowledges that she is the only one who knows the Prince's name. After admitting to Turandot that she is deeply in love with the Prince, Liu takes her own life, guarding the secret forever.

The Prince grants Turandot one more chance at freedom by divulging his name: Calaf. Moved by Liu's amorous gesture, Turandot proclaims the Prince's true name to be Love.

A romantic story for a romantic fragrance.

Introduced	1929
Price	Mid-range

LIZ CLAIBORNE

Scent Type
  Floral - Fruity
Composition
  Top Notes: *Carnation, white lily, freesia, mandarin, marigold, greens, bergamot, peach*
  Heart Notes: *Jasmine, jonquil, rose, ylang-ylang, lilac, tuberose, lily of the valley*
  Base Notes: *Sandalwood, amber, oakmoss, musk*

In 1976, American clothing designer Liz Claiborne introduced contemporary fashions to fit the way people lived. Ten years later, she created a signature fragrance that is just as comfortable and easy to wear.

A crisp, energetic blend of light florals, spirited greens and sweet fruits, the eau de toilette essence is captured in bright lacquered triangles of primary red, blue and yellow. The perfume is housed in a playfully inverted triangle-on-triangle crystalline flacon.

The scent may also be enjoyed in a variety of lotions, powders, soaps and hair products.

Introduced	1986
Price	Mid-range

LUMIÈRE

Scent Type
 Floral
Composition
 Top Notes: *Coriander, honeysuckle,
 greens, fruits, bergamot, orange blossom*
 Heart Notes: *Magnolia, acacia, tuberose,
 jasmine, lily of the valley, ylang-ylang, hyacinth*
 Base Notes: *Sandalwood, ambergris,
 tonka bean, cedarwood, moss, vetiver, musk*

From Parfums Rochas comes Lumière, a
white floral bouquet designed for the romantic
woman who is young at heart. Green fruity top
notes illuminate the light floral heart, while a
mild sandalwood base imparts a powdery finish.

 The flacon is draped in shimmering jewel
tones of sapphire, garnet and amethyst. The
luminous stopper is faceted like a fine cut jewel.

Introduced   1984
Price   Mid-range

LUTÉCE

Scent Type
 Floral - Aldehyde
Composition
 Top Notes: *Mandarin, aldehydes,
 geranium, rosewood*
 Heart Notes: *May rose, peony,
 lily of the valley, cedarwood, vetiver, orris*
 Base Notes: *Vanilla, musk, tonka bean,
 heliotrope, cinnamon*

Lutéce is a dramatic, bold fragrance from
Parfums Parquet for Houbigant.

 The dominant note in Lutéce is rose
de mai, or May rose, a rich essence grown
primarily in Grasse and Morocco. Valued for
its tenacity, it imparts voluptuous character and
longevity to this French floral composition.

Introduced   1984
Price   Mid-range

MA COLLECTION

A collection of twelve classic Jean Patou fragrances.

Famous Patrons
 Josephine Baker
 Gloria Swanson
 Duchess of Windsor
 Woolworth heiress Barbara Hutton
 Patou assistant, social journalist Elsa Maxwell
 Actress Constance Bennett
 Tennis stars Suzanne Lenglen, Helen Wills
 The society "Dolly Sisters" Rosie and Jenny
 Socialite Silvia de Castellane

Ma Collection is a reintroduction of Jean
Patou's best-loved fragrances from 1925 to
1964, twelve in total: Adieu Sagesse, Amour
Amour, Câline, Chaldée, Cocktail, Colony,
Divine Folie, L'Heure Attendue, Moment
Suprême, Normandie, Que sais-je and
Vacances. Ma Collection is a marvelous way
to try the classic French fragrances of the
legendary House of Jean Patou.

Patou's great-nephews Guy and Jean de Moüy continue the family legacy at the helm of the rue Saint-Florentin house in Paris. Jean de Moüy explains the impetus behind Ma Collection: "Our greatest desire was for these perfumes to be appreciated by the contemporary counterparts of those women who used to love wearing them; in other words, the most elegant, distinguished and also, more often than not, the most famous women in the world."

With their in-house perfumer, the master Jean Kerléo, they re-created twelve fragrances from formulas preserved by their great-uncle, the debonair Jean Patou. "This limited edition of twelve perfumes," says de Moüy, "will give lovers of all things beautiful the opportunity of inhaling the scents of a glamorous and exciting era, famous for its seductive elegance...an era in which Jean Patou became a legend in his own lifetime." The collection is now available in perfume and eau de toilette versions.

In the thirties, Patou provided a burl and glass cocktail bar in his salon to amuse the gentlemen while the women were being fitted. Along with the usual libations, an assortment of essential oils was also available so that patrons could create their own fragrances. Ma Collection takes us back to this ingenious cocktail bar tradition, reminding us of the excesses of the twenties, of the flamboyant jazz age, of aristocratic summers at the Riviera and Deauville, and of the racy Hispano Suiza automobile Patou motored throughout Europe.

Ma Collection is a thorough and thoughtful gift, an instant wardrobe of fine French perfumes. Following are highlights of each scent:

MA COLLECTION - ADIEU SAGESSE

Scent Type
  Floral - Fruity
Composition
  Top Notes: *Neroli, jonquil, lily of the valley*
  Heart Notes: *Carnation, tuberose, opopanax*
  Base Notes: *Musk, civet*

Adieu Sagesse is one of the 1925 love trilogy of fragrances, created to commemorate the moment when the body surrenders to desire. Patou envisioned the slightly spicy, tart floral for fiery redheads, though anyone can enjoy the melange of light fruity top notes artfully blended with sensual base notes.

MA COLLECTION - AMOUR AMOUR

Scent Type
  Floral - Fresh

Amour Amour was Patou's first fragrance. One of the 1925 love trilogy, he reportedly created this beguiling scent for the smoldering brunettes and dark-skinned women who made his heart beat faster. See the complete Amour Amour Profile listed earlier in this book.

MA COLLECTION - CÂLINE

Scent Type
Floral - Fresh

Composition
Top Notes: *Greens, aldehydes, mimosa, mandarin, bergamot, basil*
Heart Notes: *Iris, orange blossom, patchouli, moss, coriander*
Base Notes: *Musk, amber*

Câline debuted in 1964, the year of *My Fair Lady* and the beginning of the Beatles craze. Patou dedicated his creation to youthful women to celebrate their entrance into society. Câline is a light scent, suitable as a teenager's first serious fragrance, or for the professional woman who wants an ethereal, understated fragrance.

MA COLLECTION - CHALDÉE

Scent Type
Oriental

Composition
Top Notes: *Orange blossom, hyacinth*
Heart Notes: *Jasmine, narcissus, opopanax*
Base Notes: *Amber, spices*

Chaldée is a 1927 fragrance that derives its name from the country of Sumer in Babylonia where beautiful golden-skinned women once lived. Inspired by the new outdoor sports of the twenties, tennis and swimming, Chaldée was designed so that the richness of florals, spices and amber is brought out by the warmth of the sun. The women at Deauville and the Riviera embraced it, as did tennis champion Suzanne Lenglen.

MA COLLECTION - COCKTAIL

Scent Type
Chypre - Fruity

Composition
Top Notes: *Greens, bergamot, citrus*
Heart Notes: *Jasmine, rose*
Base Notes: *Oakmoss*

Cocktail is a refreshing splash of citrus fruits and oakmoss, a classic chypre combination. Created in 1930, it was inspired by the art of original mixing. Crisp and easy to wear, day through evening.

MA COLLECTION - COLONY

Scent Type
Chypre - Fruity

Composition
Top Notes: *Pineapple, bergamot*
Heart Notes: *Ylang-ylang, iris, carnation, opopanax*
Base Notes: *Oakmoss, leather, musk, vetiver*

Voluptuous fruits and jungle flowers are combined with woods and leathery notes to produce Colony, a chypre fragrance characterized by the marriage of fresh citrus and velvety moss. The 1938 fragrance derived its inspiration from the early colonial holdings with sun-drenched ports, lush vegetation, exotic spices and tropical sands. Colony was a favorite bon voyage gift for many a high sea journey.

MA COLLECTION - DIVINE FOLIE

Scent Type
Oriental - Ambery
Composition
Top Notes: Neroli, ylang-ylang
Heart Notes: Orange blossom, styrax, iris, rose, jasmine, vetiver
Base Notes: Musk, vanilla

Rich, intense, warm, subtle. Patou used these words to describe Divine Folie, a 1933 fragrance named after the excessive parties thrown in spite of the Depression. He wanted the perfect accompaniment to the long white satin and silk bias-cut dresses he designed to fit svelte women like a second skin. Seemingly simple, it often required two to three fittings to achieve such simplicity. Patou created the bias-cut dresses in response to Chanel's little black cocktail dress, a style he reportedly found boring.

The flowing, sensual style soared when Woolworth heiress Barbara Hutton selected one for her religious ceremony wedding gown for her first marriage to Prince Alexis Mdivani. She bought thirty-five other ensembles from Patou for her trousseau and purchased many of his designs over the years. Hutton befriended Patou and Elsa Maxwell, and the threesome attended one another's parties around the globe, from Paris to Biarritz to Morocco.

MA COLLECTION - L'HEURE ATTENDUE

Scent Type
Oriental - Spicy
Composition
Top Notes: Lily of the valley, geranium, lilac
Heart Notes: Ylang-ylang, jasmine, rose, opopanax
Base Notes: Mysore sandalwood, vanilla, patchouli

L'Heure Attendue is a 1946 fragrance crafted to celebrate the liberation of Paris from the Nazis. Formulated to reflect the happy peoples' *joie de vivre*, it is a spicy Oriental composition with an expansive, freewheeling personality.

MA COLLECTION - MOMENT SUPRÊME

Scent Type
Floral - Ambery

Composition
   Top Notes: *Lavender, geranium, clove, bergamot*
   Heart Notes: *Jasmine, rose*
   Base Notes: *Amber, spices*

Moment Suprême is a 1929 Patou concoction meant to represent Paris at its most extravagant. Like the city, the scent is enticing, sensual and sophisticated. A high society fragrance, warm and sharp.

MA COLLECTION - NORMANDIE

Scent Type
   Oriental - Ambery
Composition
   Top Notes: *Fruits*
   Heart Notes: *Carnation, jasmine, rose*
   Base Notes: *Vanilla, benzoin, oakmoss, cedarwood, woods*

The year was 1935 and the new ocean liner called the *Normandie* carried the elite of business and society on its maiden voyage from Le Havre to New York. A new Atlantic crossing speed record was set, and each passenger received Jean Patou's latest fragrance named in honor of the luxury liner. He described the fragrance as warm and determined, and packaged it in a miniature flacon surrounded by a replica of the ship. The passengers adored it.

MA COLLECTION - QUE SAIS-JE?

Scent Type
   Chypre - Fruity
Composition
   Top Notes: *Peach, apricot, orange blossom*
   Heart Notes: *Jasmine, rose, carnation, iris*
   Base Notes: *Oakmoss, patchouli*

Que sais-je? is one of Patou's 1925 love trilogy fragrances, conceived for the moment when the will hesitates. Meaning "What do I know?" in English, Que sais-je? is a light, flowery chypre blend. Patou suggested this fragrance for fair-skinned blond women, but anyone can enjoy this fresh composition.

MA COLLECTION - VACANCES

Scent Type
   Floral - Oriental
Composition
   Top Notes: *Hyacinth, hawthorn, galbanum*
   Heart Notes: *Lilac, mimosa*
   Base Notes: *Musk, woods*

Vacances debuted in 1936, the year that paid vacations came into vogue for the French. The sweet floral scent has a soft Oriental drydown. Its versatility makes it an ideal accoutrement for a sunny vacation or a day at the horse races. If it's August, this must be Deauville....

Introduced

        1925 to 1964

Price   *Mid-range*

MA GRIFFE

Scent Type
Chypre - Floral

Composition
Top Notes: *Gardenia, greens, galbanum, aldehydes, clary sage*

Heart Notes: *Jasmine, rose, sandalwood, vetiver, orris, ylang-ylang*

Base Notes: *Styrax, oakmoss, cinnamon, musk, benzoin, labdanum*

Famous Patrons
Barbara Walters

In French, *ma griffe* refers to a signature or personal stamp. Thus, couture designer Carven selected the name for her personal fragrance. Ma Griffe is a blend of earthy essences presented in brilliant green packaging. It is a timeless, easy-to-wear classic, steeped in mosses, flowers and woody balsamics.

Mme Carven founded the House of Carven in 1944. From her Paris salon at the Rond Point des Champs-Elysées, she led the way in creating haute couture especially for petite women—she herself was five feet tall. Along with her signature samba dresses, silk scarves, furs and jewelry collections, she sold fragrance creations. Though Ma Griffe was her personal scent, she also introduced other classics: Robe d'un Soir, Madame Carven, Vert et Blanc and Variations.

Introduced   *1946*

Price   *Mid-range*

MA LIBERTÉ

Scent Type
Oriental - Spicy

Composition
Top Notes: *Heliotrope, citrus*

Heart Notes: *Jasmine, rose, lavender, clove*

Base Notes: *Sandalwood, vetiver, vanilla, musk, cedarwood, patchouli, nutmeg, cinnamon*

From Jean Patou comes a haunting ambrosial fragrance invented for the woman who is free with her emotions, the expressive woman with emotional liberty.

A subtle Oriental blend, Ma Liberté begins with saucy citrus top notes followed by a courtly floral heart enhanced with spicy clove. Fragrant woods are accented with cinnamon and nutmeg to produce a sweet sensual finish, fit for Aphrodite.

For other Jean Patou fragrances, see the Profile for Ma Collection, an assortment of twelve classic scents formulated from 1925 to 1964.

Introduced   *1987*

Price   *Mid-range*

MACKIE, BOB MACKIE

Scent Type
Floral - Oriental

Composition
Top Notes: Peach, raspberry, pineapple
Heart Notes: Jasmine, rose, jonquil, orange blossom, ylang-ylang, tuberose
Base Notes: Sandalwood, vetiver, patchouli, amber, musk

Mackie is the namesake fragrance from internationally renowned designer Bob Mackie. The scent is introduced by fresh fruits, while rich white florals heighten the drama of the warm Oriental blend.

Mackie says, "A woman who wears my clothes is not afraid to be noticed." Ditto for his perfume. Mackie is the designer to the stars, the man behind some of Hollywood's most striking and alluring garments. Who could forget Cher's Oscar night attire? Classic Mackie. "Dare to be noticed—wear a Mackie Original," he says.

The sensual fragrance is captured in a multifaceted Pierre Dinand/Mackie-designed bottle, topped with a crystal stopper for added glamour and glitz. The ebony and ivory color theme reflects Mackie's love of piano. The dramatic outer package sports a brilliantly colored starburst prism.

Mackie...a glamorous fragrance for drop-dead drama.

Introduced	*1991*
Price	*High range*

MAD MOMENTS

Scent Type
Floral

Composition
Top Notes: Bergamot, galbanum, basil, tagetes, neroli, orange blossom
Heart Notes: Rose oil, rose absolute, osmanthus absolute, frangipani, geranium, jasmine, black currant bud, narcissus absolute
Base Notes: Vanilla, patchouli, amber, oakmoss, opopanax, musk, iris, benzoin

Famous Patrons
Kelly Le Brock
Jacqueline Kennedy Onassis
Diana Ross
Elsa Peretti
Imelda Marcos
Matilda (Mrs. Mario) Cuomo
Petula Clark

Mad Moments is the 1991 fragrance from creator Madeleine Mono. She says it is "for the moments that are many and the moments that are few."

The most noticeable impressions are floral, rose and chypre notes, drying down to a dramatic finale.

The packaging is appropriate for the romantic fragrance. French lead crystal bottles are nestled in boxes featuring cupids, hearts, clocks and bows. The packaging was inspired by Madeleine Mono's personal collection of Victorian-era memorabilia, particularly her decoupaged boxes. Her passion for decoupage was shared by Queen Victoria, who was an avid collector, encouraging other fashionable ladies of the era to follow suit.

Introduced 1991
Price Mid-range

MADAME ROCHAS

Scent Type
Floral - Aldehyde
Composition
Top Notes: Hyacinth, neroli, aldehydes, greens, lemon
Heart Notes: Bulgarian rose, jasmine, iris, lily of the valley, violet, orris, narcissus, tuberose
Base Notes: Amber, cedarwood, sandalwood, moss, vetiver, musk, tonka bean

Madame Rochas is a floral symphony of rich jasmine, rose and iris. The full-bodied heart is embedded in warm exotic woods. The French approach is timeless and enduring, as fine today as it was upon introduction more than three decades ago. Its personality is spicy, delicate and feminine.

Madame Rochas is presented in the signature Rochas color scheme of white, red and gold. The octagonal cylinder is a copy of an eighteenth-century cut-crystal bottle that Hélène Rochas unearthed in a Parisian antique shop. Classic design, classic fragrance, classic French.

Introduced 1960
Price Top range

MADELEINE DE MADELEINE

Scent Type
Floral
Composition
Top Notes: French tuberose absolute, French mimosa absolute, Moroccan jonquil absolute
Heart Notes: Turkish otto of rose, French jasmine absolute, Roman chamomile oil
Base Notes: Yugoslavian oakmoss absolute, French orange blossom absolute

Famous Patrons
Nancy Reagan
Brooke Shields
Mrs. Sean Connery
Kelly Le Brock
Maggie Smith
Singer Jan Chamberlin (Mrs. Mickey Rooney)
Matilda (Mrs. Mario) Cuomo

Madeleine de Madeleine is the first fragrance introduced by Madeleine Mono and is a favorite of many renowned women.

The fragrant concoction is composed of rich, long-lasting essences, such as jonquil, tuberose, mimosa and jasmine absolute. Absolutes are highly concentrated forms of essence, and Madeleine Mono uses them freely. Oakmoss and chamomile add a soothing element to the overflowing basket of florals.

The Madeleine de Madeleine scent can be purchased in a range of body care products. From its headquarters in Southampton, the company also distributes a line of well-priced cosmetics.

Introduced   1978
Price   Mid-range

MADEMOISELLE RICCI

Scent Type
  Floral - Ambery
Composition
  Top Notes: *Galbanum*
  Heart Notes: *Kazanlick rose, Florentine iris, royal lily, honeysuckle*
  Base Notes: *Patchouli, sandalwood*

Mademoiselle Ricci is an ambery floral composition, with highlights of woods and spice. A subtly sensual fragrance, it is amply refined for understated daytime sophistication.

Introduced   1965
Price   Mid-range

MAGIE NOIRE

Scent Type
  Oriental - Ambery Spicy

Composition
  Top Notes: *Hyacinth, cassie, bergamot, raspberry, galbanum*
  Heart Notes: *Jasmine, ylang-ylang, Bulgarian rose, lily of the valley, narcissus, honey, tuberose, orris*
  Base Notes: *Spices, sandalwood, ambergris, cedarwood, patchouli, oakmoss, musk, civet*

Famous Patrons
  Actress Isabella Rossellini

From Lancôme comes Magie Noire, or "black magic" in French. The spicy Oriental blend is as smooth as Far Eastern silk. Seductively understated, soothing and easy to wear, it is perfect for a little night magic.

The round bottle, designed by master bottle designer Pierre Dinand, sports a deeply indented V-shape, draped around the shoulders like a plunging neckline.

Introduced   1981
Price   High range

MAGNETIC

Scent Type
  Floral - Fruity
Composition
  Top Notes: *Mandarin, bergamot, peach, cardamom, plum, neroli*
  Heart Notes: *Jasmine, lily of the valley, tuberose, gardenia, ylang-ylang*
  Base Notes: *Sandalwood, musk, heliotrope, tonka bean, amber*

Famous Patrons
Gabriela Sabatini

The second fragrance from tennis star Gabriela Sabatini and Muelhens is Magnetic, a softer scent than her original namesake fragrance. The floral bouquet draws you in with sweet fruity top notes, like a gentle breeze whispering through an orchard in bloom.

The fragrance is packaged in a glass flacon that looks as though an invisible force, a magnetic field, has pulled it to one side. It is crowned with a red cap and housed in a fiery red and black carton.

Magnetic is a pretty daytime and warm weather fragrance, one you could easily wear on the tennis court. If only Sabatini could bottle her tennis talent for us as well.

Introduced   1993
Price   Mid-range

MAROUSSIA

Scent Type
   Floral - Oriental
Composition
   Top Notes: *Ylang-ylang, narcissus, black currant bud*
   Heart Notes: *Rose, jasmine, orange blossom, lily of the valley*
   Base Notes: *Amber, musk, vanilla, sandalwood*

From Russia with love comes Maroussia, a warm ambery Oriental blend from native son and handsome couturier Slava Zaitsev.

The sensual fragrance has mellow fruity top notes, quickly followed by a spicy floral heart that rests against a base accord of smoldering Oriental notes. The haunting melody creates a magnificent trail, or aura. Elegant and original.

Bottled in Moscow, Maroussia resides in ruby red and gold-colored flacons inspired by Russian Orthodox church domes. The fragrance is packaged in red boxes draped with an intricate print that is designed after Russian shawls and sensual Gustav Klimt paintings.

Close your eyes and imagine the snowy sleigh scenes from *Doctor Zhivago*. The romance of Russia...Maroussia.

Introduced   1992 (Europe)
Price   Mid-range

MAUD FRIZON PARFUM

Scent Type
   Floral
Composition
   Top Notes: *Lime*
   Heart Notes: *Myrtle, tuberose, jasmine, rose, tulip, gardenia*
   Base Notes: *Woods, musk*

French designer Maud Frizon offers a signature fragrance in a pleasing floral arrangement.

P.S. We've always loved her splendidly crafted, outrageous shoes.

Introduced   1985
Price   Mid-range

MICHELLE

Scent Type
    Floral
Composition
    Top Notes: Aldehydes, peach, coconut,
    greens, gardenia
    Heart Notes: Jasmine, ylang-ylang, rose,
    iris, tuberose, carnation, orchid
    Base Notes: Musk, vetiver, vanilla,
    benzoin, moss, sandalwood

Michelle is a classic floral blend from the couture firm of Cristobal Balenciaga, introduced after the designer's death. Michelle begins with snappy aldehydes and fruits. The bright mixture dissolves into a rich floral heart, supported by woody base notes with a sweet, powdery finish.

Michelle is named for Balenciaga's top model from the 1960s. Packaged in a svelte bottle designed by Pierre Dinand and clothed in hues of black, red and gold, it looks as if it's ready for a catwalk under the bright lights of haute couture.

Perfect for a Paris fashion runway, or your own personal prancing.

Introduced   1980
Price   High range

MISS BALMAIN

Scent Type
    Chypre - Floral Animalic
Composition
    Top Notes: Gardenia, coriander,
    citrus, aldehydes
    Heart Notes: Jasmine, rose,
    carnation, narcissus, orris, jonquil
    Base Notes: Castoreum, patchouli,
    oakmoss, leather, vetiver, amber

Couturier Pierre Balmain added Miss Balmain to his stable of fragrances in 1967.

Herbs and aldehydes create a jaunty, dry introduction to the chypre formula, while the addition of florals and woods lends a warm sweetness and a leathery drydown. Miss Balmain is a fragrance of proper demeanor, like a well-mannered European lady in a creamy Balmain evening gown.

Introduced   1967
Price   High range

MISS DIOR

Scent Type
   Chypre - Floral Animalic
Composition
   Top Notes: Bergamot, aldehydes, clary sage, gardenia, galbanum
   Heart Notes: Rose, jasmine, lily of the valley, carnation, orris
   Base Notes: Patchouli, oakmoss, amber, vetiver, sandalwood, leather

A classic, impeccable floral fragrance, Miss Dior was created by couturier Christian Dior.

Miss Dior was launched in 1947, the year Dior introduced his New Look. The New Look was actually a throwback to the pre-World War II years—full skirts, tiny waistlines, gloves and bare shoulders, a far cry from the despondent styles of the war years. Consumers flocked to update their wardrobes with the New Look, and they snapped up his fragrance, Miss Dior. Advertising campaigns featured the swan-like figure of a Dior model, with a flowing black bow, the re-emergence of the feminine, elegant style of the Belle Époque.

Today, the perennial French debutante Miss Dior is enjoying a resurgence, or second debut. She bows in a houndstooth-embossed clear crystal flacon, with a pristine white satin bow at her neckline. Still lovely after all these years.

Introduced   1947
Price   *High range*

MITSOUKO

Scent Type
   Chypre - Fruity
Composition
   Top Notes: Peach, bergamot, hesperides
   Heart Notes: Lilac, rose, jasmine, ylang-ylang
   Base Notes: Vetiver, amber, oakmoss, cinnamon, spices

Third generation perfumer Jacques Guerlain developed Mitsouko for women of passion, intensity, strength and introspection. Created on the eve of the Roaring Twenties, Mitsouko reflects the Far Eastern style that became the rage in the flamboyant years after World War I.

Mitsouko opens with fruity top notes of tangy bergamot and smooth, mellow peach. A lilac note blend follows, dissolving into a woody chypre drydown, redolent of vetiver, oakmoss and amber. A sensual, voluptuous fragrance, like a dark, full-bodied Cabernet Sauvignon. Enhance it with Mitsouko bath and body products.

Mitsouko means "mystery" in Japanese and was inspired by a character in the Claude Farrère novel, *La Bataille*, or *The Battle*. The story revolved around the ill-fated love of an English officer and the wife of the ship's commander, a beautiful Japanese woman named Mitsouko. Farrère had mentioned another Guerlain fragrance, Jicky, in one of his novels, so Jacques Guerlain reciprocated the honor by naming his fragrance after a Farrère character. And so Mitsouko lives on, in print and in fragrance. It remains one of the great jewels of the House of Guerlain.

Introduced   1919
Price   High range

MOLINARD DE MOLINARD

Scent Type
   Floral - Fruity
Composition
   Top Notes: Fruits, citrus,
   black currant bud, greens
   Heart Notes: Bulgarian rose,
   Grasse jasmine, narcissus, ylang-ylang
   Base Notes: Amber, Réunion Island
   vetiver, incense

From the House of Molinard comes
another classic floral bouquet, accented with
sunny top notes of fruit and citrus.

In 1849 the House of Molinard opened a
fragrance shop in Grasse, France, catering to the
wealthy clientele that came to enjoy the French
Riviera. To this day, the name of Molinard is
associated with women of fine taste and privilege.

Molinard is known for its beautiful flacons,
many created by Lalique and Baccarat. Today,
the fragrance is in a rectangular Lalique bottle,
festooned with a generous collar of frosted
glass in which are sculpted graceful female
forms. The bottle was originally designed
in 1929 for the Molinard fragrance Les Iscles
d'Or. Quite collectible.

Introduced   1980
Price   High range

MOMENTS BY PRISCILLA PRESLEY

Scent Type
   Chypre - Floral Animalic
Composition
   Top Notes: Bergamot, greens, peach, violet,
   coriander, black currant bud
   Heart Notes: Tuberose, jonquil, jasmine,
   lily of the valley, rose, ylang-ylang,
   orange blossom
   Base Notes: Vanilla, sandalwood, patchouli,
   musk, oakmoss, vetiver, amber, leather

Famous Patrons
   Priscilla Presley

Moments is a chypre floral blend from
Priscilla Presley for Muelhens. Saucy top notes
of fruits and greens smooth the way for a rosy
floral heart, blossoming on a bed of oakmoss
with Oriental accents of amber, vanilla and
patchouli. A fragrance created for special
moments...when worn properly, it can make
every moment special.

The chypre category is used to define heavy
woody floral fragrances, usually composed of
essences such as oakmoss, sandalwood, rosewood,
vetiver and patchouli. These earthy notes mix
well with intense florals such as jasmine and
rose, while citrus and fruits are added to lighten,
or lift, the fragrance. Moments is a fine
example of this fragrance category.

Stay tuned for more fragrant ventures from
multi-talented Presley.

Introduced   1990
Price   High range

MONTANA PARFUM DE PEAU

Scent Type
Chypre - Floral
Composition
    Top Notes: *Peach, plum, pepper, cassie, cardamom, greens*
    Heart Notes: *Ginger, tuberose, rose, carnation, sandalwood, jasmine, ylang-ylang*
    Base Notes: *Patchouli, amber, castoreum, vetiver, civet, musk, olibanum*

From futuristic fashion designer Claude Montana comes a sensual chypre floral melange. In the Parfum de Peau, spicy fruity top notes evolve into a dry floral heart and a long-lasting base of warm woods. Smooth, silky, sexy.

In 1993 an eau de parfum concentration was introduced to the European market with a few changes to the original formula. A rounder, richer version, it features additional Oriental base notes. Look for it packaged in shades of vibrant lapis and gold.

The fragrance is held in a stepped-spiral bottle of frosted glass, like rippling whitecaps across an undulating ocean. The weighted flacon is as smooth as a shadowy silhouette; a beautiful collector's item.

Introduced   1986
Price   High range

MOODS

Scent Type
Floral - Fresh
Composition
    Top Notes: *Greens, bergamot, lemon, fruits*
    Heart Notes: *Lily of the valley, cyclamen, orchid, jasmine, rose, carnation, orris*
    Base Notes: *Cedarwood, musk*

A frothy addition to the Krizia family of fine fragrances, Moods is a fresh floral bursting with green fruity top notes. The refreshing theme is carried through to the cool floral heart and the soft, sotto voce background. A light fragrance for lilting moods and casual days...or to keep your cool under pressure.

Look for Moods in a curved inverted step bottle, styled like a woman's Art Deco dressing table. For when you're in the mood.

Introduced   1989
Price   High range

MOSCHINO

Scent Type
Floral - Oriental
Composition
    Top Notes: *Coriander, galbanum, origan*
    Heart Notes: *Absolute of ylang-ylang, gardenia, rose, carnation, patchouli, pepper, nutmeg, sandalwood*
    Base Notes: *Musk, vanilla, amber*

Moschino was conceived by the outrageously playful Italian fashion designer Franco Moschino, who created his signature fragrance for fun, irony and revolution. A floral scent with jaunty top notes, a brisk floral heart and spicy Oriental base notes, it is ideal for the young as well as the young at heart. It is an engaging daytime scent, yet sensual enough for evening.

Moschino clearly enjoys his work. At the 1991 American sales launch at Saks New York, Moschino featured performing harlequins and clowns, and he personally selected opera singers from the renowned ranks of the Juilliard School for the Performing Arts.

The fragrance comes in flacons inspired by wine bottles and draped in ribbons featuring the Italian flag colors of red, green and white. Bath and body products are in pink and gold-colored heart-shaped containers, topped with *faux* pearls.

Introduced   1991
Price   Top range

MUST DE CARTIER

Scent Type
   Oriental - Ambery
Composition
   Top Notes: Bergamot, tangerine, lemon, aldehydes, peach, rosewood
   Heart Notes: Jasmine, leather, carnation, ylang-ylang, orris, orchid
   Base Notes: Musk, amber

Famous Patrons
   Actress Josette Banzet

Extraordinarily rich and long-lasting, Must de Cartier is a dramatic Oriental fragrance from the world-renowned jeweler, Cartier. The perfume brims with exotic florals, spices, musk and smoky amber. A splendid high-impact scent; ideal for luxurious days and opulent evening wear. The burnished topaz flacon is suspended in a gold-colored casing—a jewel in itself.

The eau de toilette is also a rich fragrance, but registers more floral and citrus notes than the perfume. The two are designed to be worn together or alone. Experiment; it's hard to go wrong when the label says Cartier.

Introduced   1981
Price   High range

MY SIN

Scent Type
   Floral - Aldehyde
Composition
   Top Notes: Aldehydes, bergamot, lemon, clary sage, neroli
   Heart Notes: Ylang-ylang, jasmine, rose, clove, orris, lily of the valley, jonquil, lilac
   Base Notes: Vanilla, vetiver, musk, cedarwood, sandalwood, tolu, styrax, civet

My Sin was introduced as part of the 1924 couture collection from the Parisian House of Lanvin, one of the first ateliers to elevate fragrance to couture standing.

The floral aldehydes impart a radiant lift, followed by sweet florals and balsamic base notes for a sinfully elegant fragrance.

My Sin is packaged in classic style in a square bottle with beveled edges, labeled in colors of black and gold. Good taste is never dated.

Introduced	*1924*
Price	*Mid-range*

MYSTÈRE

Scent Type
  Chypre - Floral Animalic
Composition
  Top Notes: *Galbanum, cascarilla, coriander, hyacinth*
  Heart Notes: *Violet, narcissus, May rose, jasmine, tuberose, lily of the valley, carnation, ylang-ylang, orris*
  Base Notes: *Cypress, oakmoss, cedarwood, musk, civet, patchouli, styrax*

Mystère is a compelling fragrance from Rochas. The mystery is revealed through the green essence of galbanum, a gum resin, and the aromatic bark scent of cascarilla, a fragrant West Indian shrub. Violet and narcissus dominate a floral bouquet that leads to foresty notes, then drifts into woody cypress and oakmoss. An earthy fragrance, full of mystery like a deep, dank forest where wood nymphs dance.

The perfume is housed in an elliptic bottle with a black geometric cap, a joint creation from bottle designers Grani and Mansau.

Introduced	*1978*
Price	*Top range*

NAHEMA

Scent Type
  Floral - Aldehyde
Composition
  Top Notes: *Peach, bergamot, greens, aldehydes*
  Heart Notes: *Rose hyacinth, Bulgarian rose, ylang-ylang, jasmine, lilac, lily of the valley*
  Base Notes: *Passion fruit, Peru balsam, benzoin, vanilla, vetiver, sandalwood*

Nahema is a charming floral aldehyde with Oriental highlights. The Guerlain fragrance unfolds with the smooth freshness of fruit, followed by a rich rose floral bouquet based on aromatic woods. An original, exotic blend; a fragrance for making grand entrances.

As with most Guerlain fragrances, Nahema began with a story. The name was inspired by a character in Scheherazade's *Thousand and One Nights.* There were twin sisters, disparate in nature. Nahema means "daughter of fire," bold and untamed. One sister was governed by passion and intensity, while the other was tender and gentle. This duality of nature in the twins served as inspiration for Guerlain's fragrance, a scent that is powerful yet delicate, sensual yet innocent.

Nahema is presented in a graceful, curvaceous bottle, a circular interplay of perfection. It is adorned with a single crystal drop—an elegant simplicity. Look for Nahema in the full range of fragrance and body products.

Introduced	*1979*
Price	*High range*

NARCISSE NOIR

Scent Type
> *Floral - Oriental*

Composition
> ***Top Notes:*** *Orange blossom, bergamot, petitgrain, lemon*
> ***Heart Notes:*** *Rose, jasmine, jonquil*
> ***Base Notes:*** *Persian black narcissus, musk, civet, sandalwood*

Created by the great perfumer Ernest Daltroff, founder of Caron, Narcisse Noir is based on the black narcissus, an exotic spring-blooming flower found in China and Persia. An Oriental blend of aromatic woods lends a lingering sensual aura to the assertive floral arrangement.

Narcisse Noir was one of the most important fragrances brought forth in 1912, an industrious year in the history of perfumery. Today it is truly an enduring, sophisticated classic. Although Daltroff died in the 1940s, his company and fragrances live on, a tribute to his talent.

Introduced   1912
Price   Mid-range

NICOLE MILLER

Scent Type
> *Aura - Floral*

Composition
> ***Top Notes:*** *Mandarin, cyclamen, freesia, ylang-ylang, peach*
> ***Heart Notes:*** *Jasmine, tuberose, rose absolute, lilac, clove, orange blossom, heliotrope*
> ***Base Notes:*** *Sandalwood, vanilla, amber, musk, tonka bean, opopanax*

"What counts to me is how good women feel wearing my clothes," says designer Nicole Miller. "I know women look good if they feel sexy. I want women to encounter this feeling with my fragrance. My fragrance is young, fun and exciting. It is fresh enough to wear every day, yet romantic and sexy, with just a touch of exotic. You know...Champagne and caviar, motorcycle and blue jeans all rolled up into one scent! Think of the best vacation you've ever been on...or a night where you felt you could dance 'til dawn. I want my scent to say 'live life to the extreme and have a great time!' Nothing stuffy or overdone, just sexy, feminine and energetic. This is the way I want women to feel every time they experience my fragrance."

Need we say more? Look for Miller's whimsical prints in silk ties, boxer shorts and more for him, and sexy, feminine, ready-to-wear for her. One of the most delightful designer lines we've seen in ages!

Worldwide manufacturer and distributor of the Nicole Miller fragrance, Riviera Concepts, says the aura-floral scent type is a new category in perfumery, and is designed to drape a fragrant silhouette over the entire body. The first encounter with Miller's fragrance is like a breeze billowing through a springtime orchard, with fruity notes of mandarin and peach. A floral heart follows, trailed by a sweet, soft accord of wooded notes. A sexy, easy-to-wear, feminine fragrance.

The charming bottle was designed in tandem by Miller and bottle designer Pierre Dinand. Reminiscent of a jewel pouch with *trompe l'oeil* lines, the "pouch of perfume" flacon is cinched at the stopper by a gold-colored cord. The theme is carried through to her Silk Bath Collection, a line of scented bath and body products.

And finally, to commemorate the launch of her first fragrance, Miller designed a brilliant silk print scarf that depicts the story behind the creation of the scent.

Introduced   1993
Price   Mid-range

NIKI DE SAINT PHALLE

Scent Type
Chypre - Floral
Composition
Top Notes: Greens, peach, bergamot, spearmint, artemisia
Heart Notes: Jasmine, carnation, rose, ylang-ylang, cedarwood, orris, patchouli
Base Notes: Oakmoss, sandalwood, leather, musk, amber

Niki de Saint Phalle is a vivid chypre floral encased in an equally vivid bottle of deepest blue, featuring entwined multicolor snakes, slithering to the neck. Playful and dramatic.

Introduced   1982
Price   High range

NINA

Scent Type
Floral
Composition
Top Notes: Bergamot, greens, basil, lemon, peach, cassie, tagetes, aldehydes
Heart Notes: Jasmine, rose, orange blossom, marigold, mimosa, violet, ylang-ylang, bay leaf, orris
Base Notes: Vetiver, sandalwood, patchouli, moss, civet, musk

A well-rounded combination of florals, fruits, greens and woods imbues this floral blend with a range of impressions—from a ribboned hillside of flowers to a ripe orchard to an herbal melange of fresh-cut fields and forests. Nina is from Nina Ricci, proof positive that the venerable French Nina Ricci company still has its touch.

Introduced   1988
Price   Mid-range

NIRO 15

Scent Type
Floral

Composition
Top Notes: *Jasmine, lily of the valley, wisteria*
Heart Notes: *Wisteria, florals*
Base Notes: *Jasmine, lily of the valley, wisteria*

Niro 15 is a floral blend from the Dallas-based Niro team of Nick Meyer and Ron Gzell. Nick Meyer describes the fragrance: "Fresh yet alluring, a scent that men widely appreciate and welcome. A fragrance favorite of many professional women." A delicate floral composition, it performs well year round but is best in spring and fall. A blend designed for royalty, it is understated and refined.

We had a delightful visit with Nick Meyer, who refrained from naming any celebrity patrons without their permission, but said, "We have more testimonials on this fragrance than Carter has pills." Now that's the kind of Texanspeak that takes us back home.

Niro 15 can be found in select specialty stores, or just call Nick. Tell him howdy for us.

Introduced 1980
Price Mid-range

NIRO 119

Scent Type
Floral

Composition
Top Notes: *Ylang-ylang, orange blossom*
Heart Notes: *Rose, jasmine*
Base Notes: *Rose, jasmine, musk*

The second fragrance from Niro is Niro 119, a woody floral composition with a dominant note of rose and a trail of musk. A dramatic, long-lasting fragrance, one you can wear to dance until dawn.

Niro partner Nick Meyer says that Niro 119 is best in cool winter weather. We concur. This is a heady, sensual scent with maximum impact.

Introduced 1983
Price Mid-range

NOCTURNES

Scent Type
Floral - Aldehyde

Composition
Top Notes: *Aldehydes, bergamot, mandarin, greens*
Heart Notes: *Rose, jasmine, ylang-ylang, tuberose, stephanotis, lily of the valley, orris, cyclamen*
Base Notes: *Vanilla, amber, musk, sandalwood, vetiver, benzoin*

Nocturnes hails from the esteemed Parisian firm of Caron. The ambrosial floral recipe is enhanced by stephanotis, a woody Greek vine that bears waxy white flowers with a full-bodied sweet scent. Sweet woods, vanilla and amber create a lingering aura.

Ever curious, we researched the word "nocturnes" and discovered quite an artistic lineage. A nocturne may be a night scene painting. Or it may be a romantic musical composition, especially for the piano, evocative of dreamy night scenes. Think of it, Caron's Nocturnes could be the perfect fragrance for a dreamy evening with a handsome artist or pianist.

Introduced	*1981*
Price	*High range*

NOIR FOR WOMEN BY PASCAL MORABITO

Scent Type
Floral
Composition
    Top Notes: *Black currant bud, mandarin*
    Heart Notes: *Jasmine*
    Base Notes: *Iris*

Designer Pascal Morabito's Noir is a floral scent with fruity top notes of black currant and sweet mandarin, embedded in a subtle spicy iris base note.

The bottle is cleverly suspended between two 24-karat gold-plated plates, fixed with rivets at each corner.

Introduced	*1993 (United States)*
Price	*Mid-range*

NORELL

Scent Type
Floral
Composition
    Top Notes: *Greens, reseda, galbanum*
    Heart Notes: *Carnation, hyacinth, rose, jasmine*
    Base Notes: *Musk, iris, sandalwood*

A classic floral fragrance, Norell zips open with snappy green notes, then does a slow dissolve to a rich, sophisticated floral heart. Spicy carnation and warm background essences create a luxurious ambiance, evocative of a Norell satin sheath.

Revlon launched the fragrance with the endorsement of American designer Norman Norell, whose philosophy was that one should always buy the best one can afford. Norell was selected in part because he was a favorite designer of Lynn Revson, wife of Revlon founding partner Charles Revson.

The glamour of Norell couture lives on in a courtly, refined fragrance that whispers of wealth.

Introduced	*1968*
Price	*High range*

NUDE

Scent Type
Floral - Aldehyde

Composition
Top Notes: Aldehydes, rose, galbanum, narcissus
Heart Notes: Jasmine, ylang-ylang, mosses
Base Notes: Musk, sandalwood, vetiver, orris

Nude is a sublime floral composition from Bill Blass for Revlon. Brisk aldehydes endow the clean fragrance with a fleeting, ethereal quality. The floral heart is blended with cool green mosses, giving way to a soft woody base with a trace of violet that is produced by the addition of orris. A refreshing, spa-like aroma.

Nude is the perfect fragrance to wear when fragrance is all you're wearing.

Introduced	1990
Price	High range

NUIT DE NOËL

Scent Type
Oriental

Composition
Top Notes: Citrus
Heart Notes: Rose, orris, jasmine, ylang-ylang
Base Notes: Sandalwood, vanilla, oakmoss

An exotic Oriental fragrance from the House of Caron, Nuit de Noël, French for

"Christmas Eve," begins with exhilarating citrus top notes, followed by a heart of rare flowers. Orris adds a subtle violet-like note to the composition, while sweet vanilla, earthy oakmoss and balsamic sandalwood are blended for a lasting aura. Nuit de Noël is a fitting fragrance for holiday galas or a romantic Christmas Eve.

Created more than seven decades ago, this classic is presented in a splendid black flacon, designed to accentuate the image of the dramatic scent.

Introduced	1922
Price	Mid-range

OBSESSION

Scent Type
Oriental - Ambery

Composition
Top Notes: Mandarin, bergamot, peach, lemon, orange blossom, greens
Heart Notes: Coriander, tagetes, armoise, jasmine, rose, cedarwood, sandalwood
Base Notes: Vanilla, amber, oakmoss, musk, civet

Obsession, the first fragrance from American designer Calvin Klein, quickly became a best-selling scent after its lavish 1985 debut. The passionate, long-lasting fragrance brims with exotic spices, vanilla and amber. Heavy, provocative, compelling. It is a distinctive fragrance, formulated to last all night and into the morning. The cognac-colored liquid is perfect for cool days and cooler evenings, but use sparingly when the heat and humidity soar.

The easy-traveling flacon is smooth and sparse, accented with amber hues tipped in gold-color, and presented in cartons of creme and navy. For particular pampering, try the Obsession bath and body products. Smooth on the golden body glistener to enhance a summer tan, or slip into a scented bath to cast your petty cares aside...and let your mind wander to your own magnificent obsession.

Introduced   1985
Price   Mid-range

ODALISQUE

Scent Type
   Oriental
Composition
   Top Notes: Citrus
   Heart Notes: White flowers
   Base Notes: Woods, spices

Famous Patrons
   Mamie Eisenhower

Odalisque is a sophisticated Oriental blend from Nettie Rosenstein, now distributed in North America by Classic Fragrances. Subtle, understated, classic.

Intrigued by the word "odalisque," we set out on a search to discover its meaning. From Turkish, we found that an odalisque, or odalisk, is a concubine in an Oriental harem. Or perhaps

Rosenstein was referring to the reclining female slaves that Matisse vividly portrayed in his sanguine paintings. Hmmm...sounds like a scent with a past....

The scent suggests crisp top notes of mandarin orange, laced with spicy lavender and iris. The heart note exudes rich Oriental white flowers, such as jasmine, set against warm woods and spices. A special item in the fragrance line is Odalisque Bubble Geleé in an authentic Champagne bottle. Indulge in a rich bath, and why not include a chilled bottle of Champagne, too?

Introduced   1950s
Price   Mid-range

OH LA LA!

Scent Type
   Oriental
Composition
   Top Notes: Raspberry, peach, mandarin, bergamot, fig leaves, muscat grape
   Heart Notes: Yellow rose, jasmine, narcissus, ylang-ylang, orange blossom, osmanthus
   Base Notes: Cinnamon, sandalwood, amber, vanilla, patchouli, tonka bean

Loris Azzaro makes a splash with Oh la la!, a festive Oriental fragrance. Azzaro says that the name connotes "wonderment, enthusiasm and joy" in French, as well as cleverly repeating his initials.

The baroque blend bubbles forth with fruity top notes and evolves into a floral heart with an Oriental base, accented by the sweet familiarity of cinnamon.

Oh la la! is held in a bottle styled like a Venetian Champagne glass, conceived by Azzaro and bottle designer Serge Mansau. The extravagance of the fragrance and bottle is carried through to the outer packaging, a design of lipstick red with gold-colored scribbles.

Salut! A fitting fragrance to toast the New Year.

Introduced	*1993 (Europe)*
Planned	*1994 or 1995 (North America)*
Price	*Top range*

OMBRE ROSE

Scent Type
Floral - Aldehyde
Composition
Top Notes: *Aldehydes, peach, rosewood, geranium*
Heart Notes: *Lily of the valley, ylang-ylang, rose, orris, sandalwood, cedarwood, vetiver*
Base Notes: *Vanilla, honey, iris, musk, cinnamon, tonka bean, heliotrope*

Ombre Rose is from Jean-Charles Brousseau, a Parisian couturier known for his expertise in millinery and accessories. The rose floral bouquet is brightened by aldehydes, peach and geranium, then warmed to a powdery finish by sweet vanilla, honey and exotic woods. Vivid

and long-lasting, Ombre Rose is an intense daytime or evening fragrance.

The perfume is presented in a burnished black hexagonal flacon, highlighted by a sculpted floral pattern. Other strengths are available in similar bottles of clear glass in bas relief. The bottle designs are based on an antique bottle from Brousseau's personal collection.

Introduced	*1981*
Price	*Mid-range*

ONE PERFECT ROSE

Scent Type
Floral
Composition
Top Notes: *Tunisian black currant bud, peach, narcissus*
Heart Notes: *Rose absolute, jasmine absolute, tuberose, gardenia*
Base Notes: *Sandalwood, vetiver, musk*

One Perfect Rose is a luxurious, sensual fragrance for the discriminating woman. Creator Georgette Mosbacher sought to capture the most perfect symbol of love in a fragrance form, and in her quest she queried the great perfumers of Europe and America. "The reply was inescapable—the same from Paris to the Vale of Kashmir—'If you seek the perfect essence of love, you seek the rose,'" says Mosbacher.

"We inhabit a frenetic world," she says, "so in our private moments, we need the solace of beautiful objects, beautiful poetry and, especially, beautiful fragrances."

And so it came to be that One Perfect Rose was centered on a feminine accord of exquisite rose absolute and fragrant white flowers, a formula created by French master perfumer Guy Roberts. The rich floral essence basks in base notes of soothing sandalwood and tenacious musk. The result is a glamorous fragrance, ideal for lunching at the Beverly Hills Bistro Garden or New York's Tavern on the Green, and a sophisticated, dramatic accent for sparkling evening wear.

The 1920s-style flacon was commissioned by England's renowned House of Boehm, masters of delicate porcelain sculptures that grace the most aristocratic homes in the world, including Buckingham Palace and the Vatican. The limited-edition one-ounce perfume flacons are hand-painted in soft hues of celadon green and accented with 24-karat gold leaf, crowned with a gilded rose stopper. A collector's item, it is priced at about $1,500. Another crystal flacon is produced by Brosse in Normandy, France, showcasing a detailed rose individually applied and polished by hand. This Gilded Rose bottle contains one ounce of perfume and is priced at about $350.

Mosbacher acquired and later sold the Swiss skin care company La Prairie, which distributed One Perfect Rose. Alas, the fragrance is not currently available from La Prairie, but look for a 1994 perfume creation from Mosbacher, as CEO of her latest cosmetic venture Exclusives, along with her sister, Lyn Paulsin. And, for inside tips on a woman's road to success, be sure to read Mosbacher's fabulous 1993 book, *Feminine Force: Release the Power Within to Create the Life You Deserve.*

Introduced	*1990*
Price	*Top range*

1000 DE JEAN PATOU

Scent Type
Floral
Composition
> **Top Notes:** *Greens, bergamot, anjelica, coriander, tarragon*
> **Heart Notes:** *Chinese osmanthus, jasmine, rose, lily of the valley, violet, iris, geranium*
> **Base Notes:** *Vetiver, patchouli, moss, sandalwood, amber, musk, civet*

Jean Kerléo, the in-house master perfumer for Jean Patou, favors the precious essence of jasmine and rose he used in abundance in 1000. The company describes the fragrance as "the essence of extravagance," a costly formula born of mostly natural ingredients.

The addition of violet, iris and aromatic woods is designed to endow the wearer with an aura of wealth, breeding and good taste. Wear it to close a multi-thousand-dollar business deal or to a thousand-dollar-a-plate fundraiser...or simply to feel like a million.

Elegant, understated and refined, it is a first class fragrance that moves gracefully through a variety of seasons and occasions. Another timeless creation from the House of Patou.

Introduced	*1972*
Price	*Top range*

ONE UNLIMITED PERFUME

Six fragrances under One name.

ONE UNLIMITED PERFUME- CAPRI

Scent Type
Floral - Fruity
Composition
Notes: Ylang-ylang, sugar plum, tuberose

ONE UNLIMITED PERFUME- EMERALD ISLE

Scent Type
Green
Composition
Notes: Greens, herbs

ONE UNLIMITED PERFUME- INDOCHINE

Scent Type
Floral - Oriental
Composition
*Top and Heart Notes: Rose,
lily of the valley, vetiver, rosemary, thyme,
olibanum, mandarin*
Base Notes: Musk, amber

ONE UNLIMITED PERFUME- MALAGA

Scent Type
Floral
Composition
*Top and Heart Notes: Jasmine, magnolia,
honeysuckle, hyacinth*
Base Notes: Musk, amber

ONE UNLIMITED PERFUME- MANDALAY

Scent Type
Floral
Composition
Top Notes: Orange blossom
Heart Notes: Lily of the valley
Base Notes: Moss

ONE UNLIMITED PERFUME- PROVENCE

Scent Type
Floral
Composition
Notes: Rose, lilac, jasmine, violet

One is a collection of six fragrances, created to reflect the exotic locales from which they draw their names and ingredients.

The One concept is that only one form of the scent is required for all uses: as a fragrance, body lotion or bath oil. It is an oil-based, alcohol-free, moisturizing perfume. The form of fragrance can be changed depending on the amount of water added. Each scent is packaged in a pump spray bottle, and all packaging is recyclable or biodegradable.

One all-over scent. One size and One price, too.

Introduced   1991
Price   Mid-range

OPIUM

Scent Type
 Oriental - Spicy
Composition
 Top Notes: *Plum, hesperides, clove, coriander, pepper, bay leaf*
 Heart Notes: *Jasmine, rose, carnation, lily of the valley, cinnamon, peach, orris*
 Base Notes: *Sandalwood, vetiver, myrrh, opopanax, labdanum, benzoin, benjamin, castoreum, amber, incense, musk, patchouli, tolu*

Famous Patrons
 Tanya Tucker
 Jerry Hall, (Mrs. Mick Jagger)

Opium is an opulent Oriental blend from French designer Yves Saint Laurent. Smoldering and dramatic, the fragrance is unveiled with spicy, fruity notes that lead to a rich bouquet of heady florals. Underscoring the composition is an exotic melange of sweet aromatic woods and incense. Opium is a distinctive fragrance, made for grand entrances and seductive evenings. So potent you'll still detect it the next morning. Beautiful in cool weather, but spritz lightly in hot humid climates, when the body lotion and powder would probably suffice.

Opium caused quite a stir with its controversial name, but the exposure helped to make it a best-selling scent. For the extravagant launch party in 1977, a tall ship, the *Peking*, was rented from the South Street Seaport Museum in New York's East Harbor, with none other than Truman Capote at the helm. The ship was dressed with banners of red, gold and purple, and the Oriental theme was carried out with a thousand-pound bronze Buddha, laden with mounds of white cattleya orchids.

Yves Saint Laurent carried the Oriental theme into the packaging design. The perfume is held in a glass vial encased in a red plastic container, inspired by Japanese *inros*. *Inros* are small lacquered cases that were once worn under kimonos on silken cords and held aromatics, herbs, perfumes and medicines.

Opium was recently recognized with a FiFi Award for perennial success from The Fragrance Foundation. Look for the fragrance in a full range of body and bath products, all packaged in deep shades of reds and golds.

Introduced   1977
Price   High range

OSCAR DE LA RENTA

Scent Type
   Floral - Ambery
Composition
   Top Notes: *Orange blossom, coriander, cascarilla, basil, peach, gardenia*
   Heart Notes: *Jasmine, tuberose, ylang-ylang, May rose, lavender, orchid*
   Base Notes: *Clove, sandalwood, amber, myrrh, lavender, patchouli, opopanax*

Famous Patrons
   Princess Margaret

In 1978, couturier Oscar de la Renta enchanted the world with his first fragrance foray. His signature scent is a delicate floral bouquet, intensely feminine, reflective of his fashion designs. The formula includes rare florals set against a backdrop of powdery woods and soft spices. De la Renta took his inspiration from his mother's flower garden, in which grew the fragrant white flowers of his native country, the Dominican Republic. The result is a very wearable fragrance, excellent for daytime and warm weather, exquisite for evening. Soft, subtle, sweet and sophisticated. A polished thoroughbred, romantically inclined.

The best-selling fragrance is featured in a curved glass flacon from bottle designer Serge Mansau, capped with a frosted glass flower and a dewdrop nestled among the petals. The fragrance garnered 1978 Fragrance Foundation Awards for best women's fragrance introduction and best women's fragrance packaging. The scent is available in a wide array of bath and body products. Our favorites are the luxurious foaming bath powder, dusting powder, soaps, body creme and a fabulous hand creme.

Introduced   1978
Price   *High range*

PALOMA PICASSO

Scent Type
   Chypre - Floral
Composition
   Top Notes: *Bergamot, neroli, lemon, ambrette*
   Heart Notes: *Jasmine, Bulgarian rose, ylang-ylang, coriander, clove*
   Base Notes: *Patchouli, vetiver, sandalwood, oakmoss, moss, amber*

From internationally acclaimed designer Paloma Picasso comes a signature fragrance as worldly, dramatic and elegant as its creator. She states: "It is a fragrance for women, not girls. It is sophisticated, not naive or innocent." She calls it jewelry for the senses.

The lush chypre scent begins with brisk citrus top notes, dissolving into rich jeweled notes of jasmine and Bulgarian rose, poised against layers of spices and woods, warm ambers, earthy oakmoss and exotic sandalwood. Presented in a flawless crystal ball, the perfume is wreathed by frosted French glass. It is packaged in Paloma's signature Florentine red, contrasted by matte black.

Paloma was born into a world of creativity, the daughter of artist Pablo Picasso and Francoise Gilot. She was christened Paloma, meaning "dove" in Spanish, after her father's dove, which was the symbol of the 1949 Peace Congress. She expresses her artistic genius in myriad ways, from her jewelry designs for Tiffany to her china and crystal creations for Villeroy & Boch.

She says: "As jewelry can please the eye and the hand, so fragrance can please the senses ...revealing new sensory delights layer by layer. It is an intimate ornament that becomes part of your identity...a part of the mosaic of your life."

Her philosophy is evident throughout her work. Even some of the bath and body products leave a jewel-like sheen on the skin—the powder is flecked with gold-colored crystals.

Paloma Picasso: an elegant, assertive designer in her own right.

Introduced   1984
Price   High range

PANTHÈRE

Scent Type
  Floral - Ambery
Composition
  Top Notes: *Ginger, pepper, black currant bud, peach, coriander, plum*
  Heart Notes: *Jasmine, narcissus, rose, tuberose, gardenia, heliotrope, carnation, ylang-ylang*
  Base Notes: *Musk, sandalwood, patchouli, amber, oakmoss, cedarwood, vanilla, tonka bean*

The second women's fragrance from Cartier is a bewitching fragrance in a stunning package. Panthère is the fragrance counterpart to the sleek signature panther jewelry for which Cartier has been famous throughout the decades. For the Panthère perfume, lavish essences of florals, fruits, spices and woods are blended to create an expressive, sensual scent. Panthère eau de toilette is a lighter, fresher version of the perfume, with additional top notes of lemon, mandarin and grapefruit, while lily of the valley lightens the heart note.

The bottle, from Pochet et du Courval, is designed in the style of Cartier jewelry. Twin panthers perch on either side of the round flacon. An exquisite presentation, it is also one of the more affordable Cartier "jewels."

Introduced   1988
Price   High range

PARFUM D'HERMÈS

Scent Type
  Semi-Oriental
Composition
  Top Notes: *Aldehydes, bergamot, galbanum, hyacinth*
  Heart Notes: *Egyptian jasmine, Florentine iris, Nossi-bè ylang-ylang, Bulgarian rose, labdanum*
  Base Notes: *Cedarwood, vetiver, sandalwood, amber, spices, incense, myrrh, vanilla*

Parfum d'Hermès is a semi-Oriental fragrance from Hermès, rich, warm and sensuous, with lush florals and exotic base notes; a refined day-to-evening fragrance with a proper pedigree.

Encased in a graceful oval bottle, the scent sports a delicate piece of metal reminiscent of a stirrup strap. Packaged in red, Parfum d'Hermès is a delightful addition to any fragrance wardrobe.

Introduced	*1984*
Price	*Top range*

PARFUM SACRÉ

Scent Type
Oriental - Spicy
Composition
Top Notes: *Pepper, cinnamon, coriander, clove*
Heart Notes: *Rose, jasmine, orange blossom, mimosa*
Base Notes: *Myrrh, musk, amber, vanilla*

If the Parfum Sacré fragrance smells familiar, it is—Parfum Sacré is a classic scent that has been reintroduced by Caron. It is based on the original Caron Or et Noir fragrance, or "gold and black."

Parfum Sacré is composed of sacred essences, beginning with spicy top notes and giving way to a rich floral center, embedded in a precious blend of amber, musk, myrrh and vanilla—a warm, long-lasting composition. Elegant and feminine, it is a timeless floral fragrance.

Introduced	*1992*
Price	*High range*

PARIS

Scent Type
Floral
Composition
Top Notes: *Rose petals, orange blossom, mimosa, cassia, hawthorn, nasturtium, bergamot, greens, hyacinth*
Heart Notes: *Rose, violet leaves, jasmine, orris, ylang-ylang, lily of the valley, lily, linden blossom*
Base Notes: *Sandalwood, amber, musk, moss, iris, cedarwood, heliotrope*

In this floral bouquet, Yves Saint Laurent has captured the very essence of the grand city of Paris.

Paris is a profuse bundle of flowers, with rich sweet rose top notes and heady floral heart notes, set against warm woods and moss. An abundance of femininity sparkles in its spirit and soul. An extravagant, radiant fragrance.

Think of Paris in the springtime, the Place Vendôme, the rue de Rivoli, the Louvre, the Musee D'Orsay...we love it. Look for Paris attired in—what else?—rose petal pink and chic jet black.

Introduced	*1984*
Price	*Mid-range*

PARURE

Scent Type
Chypre - Floral Animalic
Composition
*Top Notes: Plum, bergamot, fruits,
hesperides, greens
Heart Notes: Rose, lilac, jasmine,
lily of the valley, jonquil, narcissus, orris
Base Notes: Oakmoss, patchouli,
spices, amber, leather*

Parure is a sophisticated melange from fifth-generation Guerlain perfumer Jean-Paul Guerlain. An unaffected blend of chypre, fruit and floral notes results in a lightly balanced, elegant scent. Distinctly feminine. Guerlain says it is "for an aesthetic, discerning woman, constantly in search of quality and truth."

Parure is French for "adornment," referring to precious luxuries. Where Guerlain created Chamade for the modern liberated woman, and Chant d'Arômes for youthful innocence, Parure was designed for the woman who is at ease with herself and appreciates the luxuries her life holds.

Introduced   1975
Price   Mid-range

PASSION

Scent Type
Floral
Composition
*Top and Heart Notes: Jasmine, tuberose
Base Notes: Vanilla*

Two years in the making, this warm, sensual fragrance was developed in Grasse, France, by Annick Goutal. Not to be confused with her own Gardénia Passion, nor with Elizabeth Taylor's Passion.

The heady combination of jasmine and tuberose is balanced by a tenacious drydown note of vanilla. A long-lasting, intensely feminine fragrance, Passion is appropriately named according to the Victorian language of flowers. White jasmine meant amiability, yellow jasmine conveyed grace and elegance, while Spanish jasmine denoted sensuality. And tuberose? Dangerous pleasures. A passionate, dangerous abundance of significant floral essences.

Introduced   1986
Price   High range

PAVLOVA

Scent Type
Floral

Composition

> **Top Notes:** *Hyacinth, bergamot, galbanum, black currant bud*
> **Heart Notes:** *Rose, jasmine, tuberose, orchid, narcissus, orris*
> **Base Notes:** *Sandalwood, musk, amber, cedarwood, benzoin, moss*

Famous Patrons

> *Ballerina Anna Pavlova*

A tender, classic floral, Pavlova was created in honor of the glorious Russian ballerina Anna Pavlova, who lived from 1885 to 1931. Fragrance is a beautiful part of Russian ballet history. Legend has it that each ballerina was assigned a scent, a fragrance to be worn in extravagance all over the body and hair. Thus the ballet was an experience not only in vision and sound, but also in smell. Patrons could close their eyes and imagine gliding through a flower garden, so sweet was the symphony of fragrance from the dancers. The Russian-born choreographer George Balanchine continued the tradition with the American Ballet Theater in New York City, which he founded in 1933.

Pavlova is presented in dramatic black flacons, enhanced by delicate pink flowers that entwine the bottles. Others are of clear glass, featuring a graceful swan. Long after the fragrance is finished, the bottles will beautify any dressing table. They are as lovely as the fragrance, a delicate floral scent, fresh, soft, romantic and understated.

Introduced	*1922*
Price	*Mid-range*

PHEROMONE

Scent Type

> *Green*

Composition

> **Top Notes:** *Greens, spices*
> **Heart Notes:** *Florals, jasmine*
> **Base Notes:** *Exotic woods, bark, seeds, wine resins, wild grasses*

Famous Patrons

> *Cher*
> *Actress Josette Banzet*

From Marilyn Miglin comes a precious fragrance called Pheromone. The company says the word "pheromone" means, "an organic scent signal used to communicate. From the Greek *pherein* (to carry) and *hormon* (to excite)."

When Marilyn Miglin decided to create a fragrance for her salon clientele, she searched the world for just the right formula. She journeyed to New York, Grasse, and finally Egypt, where she had ancient hieroglyphs translated to find recipes for perfume compounds. Says Miglin, "Ancient civilizations actually used fragrance to evoke behavioral responses." The ancient recipes were etched on stone temple walls, formulas for high priests and royalty. "The recipes we found contained ancient secrets that made perfume intriguing, long-lasting and communicative," reports Miglin. Thus, Pheromone was developed, a modern blend of 179 rare essences with a dominant green note.

Pheromone is also available in a body and bath line. Use the Fluid Gold body moisturizer and Gold Dust body powder to achieve shimmering golden highlights on the skin. Perfect for our wintertime cruises, no?

News Flash: We just received word that Marilyn Miglin has a new fragrance in the works for 1994 or 1995, called Untouchable. Stay tuned.

Introduced   1980
Price   Top range

POISON

Scent Type
Floral - Ambery
Composition
Top Notes: *Coriander, plum, pimento, anise, rosewood*
Heart Notes: *Rose, tuberose, orange blossom, honey, cinnamon, wild berries, cistus, labdanum, carnation, jasmine*
Base Notes: *Sandalwood, cedarwood, vetiver, musk, vanilla, heliotrope, opopanax*

Famous Patrons
Ms. Olympia bodybuilder Lenda Murray

The introduction of Poison rocked the fragrance world in 1986 with its controversial name and powerful aroma. Spicy, strong and sensual, the long-lasting concoction from the House of Christian Dior is rife with the scent of exotic florals, fruits and woods. We detect a hint of raspberry, along with cassis, or black currant bud, with a distinct Oriental drydown.

The scent is passionately presented in a deep violet flacon and packaged in hues of emerald and royal purple. A rich, opulent scent, ideal for cold winters and hot, hot evenings.

For a fresh green twist on Poison, try the 1994 introduction called Tendre Poison from Christian Dior.

Introduced   1986
Price   High range

PRÉLUDE

Scent Type
Oriental - Spicy
Composition
Top Notes: *Aldehydes, bergamot, orange, pimento*
Heart Notes: *Carnation, jasmine, rose, ylang-ylang, orchid, cinnamon*
Base Notes: *Amber, vanilla, patchouli, civet, benzoin, tolu, olibanum*

From the celebrated couturier Balenciaga comes Prélude, a spicy Oriental blend with a touch of youthful insouciance.

Fruity aldehydic top notes meld with a spicy floral heart and a soothing Oriental base of balsamic and animal notes. The juice is held in curvaceous bottles topped in hues of red and gold, created by bottle designer Pierre Dinand.

Prélude takes its name from the world of music and is meant to suggest anticipation. We can't help but wonder...anticipation of what? That part we leave to you.

Introduced   1982
Price   *High range*

PRIVATE COLLECTION

Scent Type
Chypre - Green
Composition
Top Notes: *Greens, hyacinth, citrus*
Heart Notes: *Jasmine, narcissus, rose, pine, reseda*
Base Notes: *Oakmoss, cedarwood, amber, musk*

Famous Patrons
Princess Grace

Private Collection is a fresh green chypre composition that was Estée Lauder's private perfume. As the story is told, Lauder often tried out a variety of scents while she was creating a new fragrance for her company. Naturally, she had a cache of personal favorites. When complimented on her scent one time, she was asked what it was; she replied that it was from her private collection. Soon the word spread, and customers began asking for "private collection" at Lauder counters. Estée Lauder accommodated them, and thus was born Private Collection.

Introduced   1973
Price   *Mid-range*

QUADRILLE

Scent Type
Floral
Composition
Top Notes: *Plum, peach, lemon*
Heart Notes: *Jasmine, clove, cardamom*
Base Notes: *Amber, musk*

Quadrille is a classic 1950s fragrance from Spanish couturier Cristobal Balenciaga. The floral composition opens with a splash of summer fruits. Rich jasmine is blended with the spicy seductiveness of clove, warmed by the mystery of musk and amber.

An enchanting experience...wear it for an evening of flamenco dancing.

Introduced   1955
Price   *High range*

QUARTZ

Scent Type
Floral - Fruity
Composition
Top Notes: *Peach, hyacinth, cassie*
Heart Notes: *Jasmine, rose, carnation, orris, melon*
Base Notes: *Sandalwood, musk, amber, moss, benzoin, cedarwood*

Quartz is a fruity floral from Molyneux. Peach and melon impart a fresh twist to the floral bouquet, which dries down to a mossy powdery finish. The classic fragrance is presented in smart packaging in shades of black and gold.

The House of Molyneux was founded by the British-born Captain Edward Molyneux in Paris in 1919, and became known for flowing, understated gowns and accompanying fragrances such as Vivre, Fête and Initiation. Christian Dior, Pierre Balmain and other young couturiers trained under Molyneux before he passed control to his nephew in 1967. He died in 1974 in Monte Carlo, but his influence on the world of fashion and fragrance lives on.

Introduced   1978
Price   Mid-range

QUELQUES FLEURS L'ORIGINAL

Scent Type
   Floral
Composition
   Top Notes: *Greens, bergamot, orange blossom, lemon, tarragon*
   Heart Notes: *Rose, jasmine, tuberose, lily of the valley, ylang-ylang, carnation, heliotrope, orchid, orris*
   Base Notes: *Sandalwood, oakmoss, amber, musk, tonka bean, civet*

Famous Patrons
   Sarah Bernhardt
   Actress Josette Banzet

One of the most important fragrances in history, Quelques Fleurs was the first true multi-floral, reportedly utilizing 313 different floral essences. Its development changed the approach to perfumery in the early 1900s, from subtle single florals to radiant multi-floral bouquets, and firmly established Paris as the foremost city of perfumery.

In 1987, Houbigant responded to consumer requests and reintroduced the fragrance— a devastatingly feminine scent, classic and sophisticated, evocative of acres of intoxicating flowers. Beautiful for daytime into evening, with fresh green top notes amid expansive florals and ambery woods. A classic revisited.

Introduced   1912
Reintroduced   1987
Price   Top range

RAFFINÉE

Scent Type
   Floral - Oriental
Composition
   Top Notes: *Orange blossom, bergamot, plum, clary sage*
   Heart Notes: *Osmanthus, jasmine, tuberose, ylang-ylang, rose, carnation, orchid*
   Base Notes: *Sandalwood, spices, vetiver, cinnamon, vanilla, musk*

Raffinée is a dramatic, opulent Oriental blend, rich and luxurious in the Houbigant tradition. In French the name refers to a refined elegance, an appropriate description.

A harmony of fruits and florals introduces the fragrance, followed by a full-bodied floral bouquet set against a warm backdrop of sweet spices, woods and amber. Perfect for sophisticated day wear and black-tie evenings.

Continuing the top-drawer theme, Raffinée is presented in royal shades of lacquered red and gold.

Introduced   1982
Price   High range

REALITIES

Scent Type
  Floral - Oriental
Composition
  Top Notes: *Bergamot, chamomile, sage, osmanthus*
  Heart Notes: *Bulgarian rose, jasmine, white lily, carnation, freesia*
  Base Notes: *Vanilla, amber, sandalwood, peach*

Realities is the second fragrance launched by Liz Claiborne Cosmetics. Fresh top notes of herbs and bergamot are blended with a light floral accord, backed up by soft Oriental base notes blended with gentle peach. Realities is an easy-to-wear fragrance for daytime, office and casual time; comfortable and relaxing.

A Claiborne spokesperson says that "Realities celebrates the intimacy and reality of a woman's life as she and her family truly live it," and that research showed that most women were "happy and content with their lives; fantasy escape was not for them." As the Claiborne ad says, "Reality is the best fantasy of all."

Realities comes in an artful flacon—a trio of stacked cubes, with the top cube as the cap, colored in teal. Very clean, very crisp—very Liz Claiborne.

Introduced   1990
Price   Mid-range

REALM

Scent Type
  Oriental
Composition
  Top Notes: *Sicilian mandarin, Italian cassia, Egyptian tagetes*
  Heart Notes: *Water lily, living peony*
  Base Notes: *Honey, vanilla*

Realm is a rich Oriental blend, and the first fragrance to include synthetic human pheromones.

Scientists have long acknowledged the existence of animal pheromones, the source of a kind of sixth sense in the animal world. Animals secrete a substance that affects the behavior of others of the same species. From the Greek *pherein* and *hormon*, pheromone literally means "to carry excitement." Animals use this silent language to send messages about danger, food sources, death, territorial boundaries or sexual readiness.

Turning to the human species, neuroscientists found a small receptacle in the nose called the vomeronasal organ, or VNO. It seems that the VNO might be a human pheromone receiver independent of our sense of smell, a type of sixth sense. Erox Corporation scientists conducted tests with synthetic human pheromones and reported that test subjects experienced feelings of "warmth, comfort, happiness and ease." As a result, these synthetic pheromones are placed at the heart of the Realm fragrance.

Realm is the first fragrance creation from the Erox Corporation. They comment: "We can create, for the first time, a whole new category of fragrance products with human pheromones. This marriage of technology with fine fragrances is a genuine breakthrough for the industry, because these perfumes can totally engage the senses."

Realm is packaged in a sleek modern flacon from Pierre Dinand and is currently available only by mail order, though plans are in place for future exclusive distribution.

While we can't vouch for the pheromonal effectiveness of Realm, it is a fine fragrance from an accomplished team of experts, and an exciting concept from the realm of science.

Introduced   1993
Price   Mid-range

RED

Scent Type
   Floral - Aldehyde
Composition
   Top Notes: *Osmanthus, ylang-ylang, orange blossom, peach, bergamot, spices, cassie, tagetes, hyacinth, cardamom, aldehydes*
   Heart Notes: *Jasmine, carnation, Bulgarian rose, marigold, May rose, gardenia, tuberose, orris, lily of the valley*
   Base Notes: *Amber, musk, patchouli, sandalwood, oakmoss, vetiver, tonka bean, cedarwood, vanilla, labdanum*

Red is a soft, sophisticated scent from Giorgio Beverly Hills. Each drop contains a blend of 692 ingredients—just a sampling is noted above. Red unfolds with green and fruity top notes that include peach and bergamot, aided by sweet orange blossom and ylang-ylang. A rich, yet subtle floral bouquet rests at the heart of the composition, which dissolves into a lingering accord of fragrant woods.

The fragrance, body and bath collection is clothed in distinctive red and purple packaging. We like the super moisturizing body creme with the ruby red capsules that melt into the skin.

Red is the sophisticated sister of Giorgio; quieter and more refined. Red is a fitting fragrance for career wear, from day into evening.

Introduced   1989
Price   Mid-range

RED DOOR

Scent Type
  Floral - Ambery

Composition
  Top Notes: *Red roses, ylang-ylang, peach, plum*
  Heart Notes: *Winter Oriental orchid, jasmine, lily of the valley, Moroccan orange blossom, forest lilies, wild violets, freesia, tuberose, rose*
  Base Notes: *Vetiver, honey, cedarwood, sandalwood, amber, heliotrope, musk, benzoin*

Red Door takes its name from Elizabeth Arden's world-famous spas, the Red Doors. This lovely floral opens with an accord of fruits and red roses, followed by a floral bouquet featuring an Oriental orchid that blooms only in winter. Warm drydown notes of woods and amber round out the composition. Red Door is an enduring floral fragrance, suitable for high tea or career wear.

Red Door can be found at fine department stores, in an archway-shaped bottle topped with a cap of Red Door red.

It's like opening a door to a bouquet of heavenly red roses.

Introduced   1989
Price   Mid-range

REVERIE

Scent Type
  Green

Composition
  Notes: *Green botanicals, herbs*

Famous Patrons
  Princess Diana of Wales

Fine fragrance purveyor William Owen introduced Reverie in 1993. Of it, he says, "Reverie is nature-identical, capturing the elusive and fleeting essence of green and living botanicals, always fresh and bright." A dreamy, fresh scent for daytime and active wear. Ah, we feel as though we were back in Britain, punting along the River Cam through Cambridge, in a narrow wooden boat with an Oxford man at the helm, an English spring breeze rustling our lace petticoats....

Reverie comes in plain and jewel-encrusted flacons, designed by Owen. To reflect the green notes of the fragrance, Reverie is draped with Swarovski Viennese crystals in hues of emerald and light rose, brilliantly set in 22-karat gold.

Introduced   1993
Price   Mid- to High range

RIVE GAUCHE

Scent Type
    Floral - Aldehyde
Composition
    Top Notes: Aldehydes, bergamot,
    greens, peach
    Heart Notes: Magnolia, jasmine,
    gardenia, geranium, iris, ylang-ylang,
    rose, lily of the valley
    Base Notes: Mysore sandalwood, Haitian
    vetiver, tonka bean, musk, moss, amber

Famous Patrons
    Woolworth heiress Barbara Hutton

From designer Yves Saint Laurent, Rive Gauche is a profusion of delicate, sweet white flowers, placed against a backdrop of woods and moss, all briskly introduced with ephemeral aldehydic notes. The result is a light, pleasing symphony.

Look for the complete line of Rive Gauche fragrance and body care products, packaged in distinctive midnight blue and black.

Introduced   1971
Price   High range

ROMA

Scent Type
    Oriental - Ambery
Composition
    Top Notes: Sicilian bergamot, black
    currant bud, mint
    Heart Notes: Rose, jasmine, lily of
    the valley, carnation
    Base Notes: Civet, castor, Singapore
    patchouli, Yugoslavian oakmoss,
    and balsamo, consisting of North African
    myrrh, Siamese ambergris, vanilla

Created by the renowned Italian fashion designer Laura Biagiotti, Roma is her love letter to her native city of Rome. Roma begins with the freshness of Sicilian bergamot, followed by an opulent floral bouquet. But Biagiotti's real secret behind this long-lasting fragrance lies in the discreet background notes of spicy balsamo, a blend that she says is based on a "seductive fragrance favored by women in ancient Rome." A chameleon-like spicy fragrance, Roma moves easily from casual daytime use to career and evening wear.

Subtle and complex, Roma was designed as a scent of eternal romance. The exquisite bottle was inspired by ancient Roman columns, and the outer packaging is evocative of richly veined Italian marble. A fragrant tribute to a proud and ancient city.

Introduced   1987
Price   Mid-range

ROMEO GIGLI

Scent Type
Floral - Fruity

Composition
Top Notes: *Sicilian lime, bergamot, mandarin, mango, black currant bud*
Heart Notes: *Orange blossom, rose, wild lily of the valley, jasmine, white carnation*
Base Notes: *Incense, iris, sandalwood*

The signature fragrance from noted Italian designer Romeo Gigli is a fresh floral with fruit accents. It opens with zesty top notes, like a basket of ripe Mediterranean fruit. Following is an intoxicating bouquet of just-picked flowers, underscored by spicy iris, incense and soft sandalwood.

Gigli fashioned the exquisite perfume bottle after his own antique inkwell. The slender neckline slopes to a wide round base and the pointed cap sports a frosted squiggle, like a futuristic hat.

Introduced   *1990*
Price   *High range*

ROSE ABSOLUE

Scent Type
Floral

Composition
Notes: *May rose, Turkish rose, Bulgarian rose, Damascus rose, Egyptian rose, Moroccan rose*

An international cornucopia of roses was gathered for this brilliant, fragrant exaltation from Annick Goutal. It is a superbly feminine fragrance celebrating the rose—the queen of flowers.

The scent of the rose is one of nature's most powerfully sensual aromas, and the rose is one of the most coveted flowers in history. In old Persia, the Sultan slept on a mattress filled with rose petals. Fountains of rose water adorned tables at feasts, and rose petals were often strewn among party guests. In the Victorian language of flowers, roses are the symbol of love. White roses represent purity and spiritual love; red roses mean true love; cabbage roses are ambassadors of love; a single rose denotes simplicity; burgundy roses mean unconscious beauty. But beware the yellow rose, for it represents decreasing love and infidelity.

Introduced   *1986*
Price   *Top range*

ROSE CARDIN

Scent Type
Floral - Oriental

Composition
Top Notes: *Moroccan tarragon, clove, nutmeg, coriander, rosewood*
Heart Notes: *Spicy rose, jasmine, peach, apricot, iris, lily of the valley, ylang-ylang, carnation*
Base Notes: *Honey, sandalwood, vanilla, amber, patchouli, musk*

Rose Cardin is a floral Oriental composition from Paris couturier Pierre Cardin. The fragrance begins with seductive spices, then develops into a melange of rich florals and smooth fruits. Chypre notes of patchouli create a finale that lingers on the skin with warm Oriental touches of honey, sandalwood, vanilla and musk.

Pierre Cardin worked with Dior and Schiaparelli before opening his own atelier. Multifaceted, he is known for popularizing such fashions as mini-dresses, bubble dresses and astronaut suits. He introduced the first-ever men's couture collection in 1960, and he applies his design skills to theater costumes, autos, home furnishings, real estate developments and of course, fragrance.

The perfume is housed in a columnar opaque glass container in passionate hues of rose and violet. Rose Cardin is pure Cardin, pure elegance.

Introduced   1992
Price   Mid-range

ROYAL SECRET

Scent Type
   Oriental
Composition
   Top Notes: Citrus, African orange
   Heart Notes: Bulgarian rose, jasmine
   Base Notes: Sandalwood, musk, myrrh

Germaine Monteil introduced Royal Secret nearly six decades ago, at a time when royal families still had secrets. The thirties were the height of fascination with all things Oriental, and Royal Secret reflects this attitude.

The fiery creation opens with fresh citrus notes, then combines a classic French heart of jasmine and rose with exotic base notes of sandalwood, musk and myrrh. Royal Secret...as powerful today as it was in 1935.

Introduced   1935
Price   Mid-range

RUMBA

Scent Type
   Chypre - Floral Animalic
Composition
   Top Notes: Mirabelle plum, peach, orange blossom, raspberry
   Heart Notes: Magnolia, tuberose, orchid, gardenia, jasmine, carnation, heliotrope, honey, lily of the valley
   Base Notes: Amber, oakmoss, vanilla, sandalwood, cedarwood, tonka bean, musk, styrax

Deep, sensual and opulent, this rich Balenciaga fragrance begins with spirited fruity notes, giving way to exotic florals based in sweet amber and vanilla. The rumba is a dance of Cuban-African origin, based on strong rhythmic movement. Like the dance, Rumba is not for the faint of heart but for those who want to dance until dawn and live life to the fullest.

It is housed in a dramatic bottle with horizontal bevels, like a staircase leading to the opalescent glass stopper. Look for Rumba in the deep red and black packages...and we'll see you on the dance floor.

Introduced   1989
Price   High range

SAFARI

Scent Type
   Floral - Green
Composition
   Top Notes: Tagetes, orange de Indes, hyacinth, black currant bud, jonquil, mandarin, galbanum
   Heart Notes: Italian jasmine, orange blossom, orris, genet, May rose, narcisse de Montagne
   Base Notes: Sandalwood, cedarwood, vetiver, patchouli, amber

Famous Patrons
   Actress Josette Banzet

Safari is rich in greens and florals; a fragrance designed as part of the Ralph Lauren lifestyle for Cosmair, Inc. Vigorous green notes accompany floral, citrus and woody essences in the scent that was created for women of independent and adventurous spirit. Safari is an elegant selection for warm weather, career and casually elegant evening wear.

The soft, sensual perfume is presented in curved flacons of hand-cut crystal, reminiscent of a gentle bygone era. Etched sterling silver hinged caps with tortoise shell accents complete the accoutrements a traveler might pack for an African safari. Imagine Meryl Streep in *Out of Africa.* Safari won two Fragrance Foundation Awards in 1990, for the most successful women's fragrance introduction in a limited category, and for the best national advertising TV campaign for a women's fragrance.

Lauren designed a whole world of products around the Safari theme, "a world without boundaries." He says: "I see the Safari woman as an expression of the dreams and yearnings that women have for adventure, romance and intrigue. This elegant woman represents a state of mind in which she is surrounded by luxury, yet is always at ease and comfortable with where she is and who she is. She appreciates the finest in art, clothing and her surroundings, and travels the world in search of experiences that interest and stimulate her." Oh, yes...that's us!

To complement Safari fragrances, Lauren offers a line of rich bath and body products called Safari Climate Response. The perfumed body creme sparkles on the skin; it is a richer version of the shimmering gold-colored veil found in the Safari Climate Response Body Lotion. For a real Ralph Lauren immersion, visit his boutiques in New York and on Beverly Hills' Rodeo Drive—makes us want to start packing for a well-heeled safari.

Lauren is also involved in many philanthropic activities. Through personal donations and fundraising efforts, he recently launched the Nina Hyde Center for Breast Cancer Research

at Georgetown University, named in honor of
the late Washington Post fashion editor. He
also finds time to support pediatric cancer
research and a host of children's charities.

Introduced   *1990*
Price   *Top range*

SALVADOR DALI

Scent Type
     Floral - Aldehyde
Composition
     Top Notes: *Aldehydes, mandarin,*
     bergamot, basil, greens
     Heart Notes: *Jasmine, lily of the valley,*
     tuberose, rose, narcissus, orris
     Base Notes: *Cedarwood, amber,*
     vanilla, sandalwood, musk, benzoin

Famous Patrons
     Princess Caroline of Monaco

Artist Salvador Dali lends his name to a
fragrance as surreal as his paintings.

Bright aldehydic notes spill forth from
the rich floral bouquet, while soft Oriental base
notes add ambery verve. Splash it on for a busy
day at the office or a slow stroll though your
favorite museum.

The juice is poured into a signed flacon
that mimics a partial visage. The humorous
bottle is crafted in the shape of voluptuous lips,
over which rests a nose-shaped stopper. We
had to buy this one just for the bottle.

Introduced   *1983*
Price   *High range*

SAMSARA

Scent Type
     Floral - Oriental
Composition
     Top Notes: *Bergamot, peach, lemon, greens*
     Heart Notes: *Jasmine, orris absolute,*
     ylang-ylang, rose, narcissus, santal
     Base Notes: *Amber, vanilla, sandalwood,*
     tonka bean, musk

A 1989 addition to the Guerlain fragrance
legend, Samsara is a tantalizing Oriental blend
with exotic floral accents. The name is a
Sanskrit word that signifies an infinite cycle
of births and rebirths, repeated until perfection
or nirvana is attained.

The rich fragrance is made using almost
entirely natural ingredients. Dominant notes
of jasmine, rose and ylang-ylang mingle with
balsamic sandalwood and vanilla, while the seed
of tonka bean adds a gingerbread-like aroma.
Many of the ingredients used in Samsara are
also used in aromatherapy to impart a sense
of serenity. The result is a warm, beguiling
fragrance, sensual and long-lasting.

Samsara was eleven years in the making.
Perfection was essential for creator Jean-Paul
Guerlain because the fragrance is a tribute to
the woman he loves. Inspired by her grace and
confidence, radiance and generosity, he sought
a feminine fragrance to honor her spiritual and

physical beauty. "I was but the stonemason; she was the architect," he says, and he still mixes a special version by hand just for her.

Jean-Paul Guerlain travels the Earth in search of the highest-quality ingredients for Guerlain perfumes. The company lists the sacred components they search out: "Jasmine, rose and tuberose from Mediterranean shores; sandalwood, cinnamon and bois de rose from Southeast Asia; geranium, verbena and palmarosa from Madagascar; bergamot from Calabria; vetiver from Réunion Island; and the essences of ylang-ylang and eucalyptus from the South Pacific." Indeed, Guerlain fragrances contain the essences of the world—or rather, the best of its essence.

Samsara comes in a perfume flacon inspired by ancient Asian artifacts. Colored deep red, the sacred color, it features lotus-like lines of elegant simplicity and is accented with a gold-colored sash and smooth cap. Graceful upturned edges remind us of pagodas that dot the verdant hills lining the shores of Taiwan, Korea and Japan.

Introduced   1989
Price   High range

SCAASI

Scent Type
   Floral
Composition
   Top Notes: Apricot, mandarin, rose, coriander, orange blossom, bergamot, greens
   Heart Notes: Narcissus, living tuberose, jasmine, carnation, violet, rose, ylang-ylang, gardenia
   Base Notes: Amber, oakmoss, sandalwood, vetiver, musk, vanilla, civet

Scaasi is a floral bouquet from fashion designer Arnold Scaasi. Scintillating fruits are mixed with expansive florals, woods and vanilla.

Scaasi is sumptuously packaged in satin jewel tones.

Introduced   1989
Price   High range

SCHERRER 2

Scent Type
   Floral - Aldehyde
Composition
   Top Notes: Aldehydes, peach, mandarin, pineapple, anise, greens, bergamot
   Heart Notes: Rose, lily of the valley, jasmine, orris, lily, honey, tuberose
   Base Notes: Vanilla, sandalwood, amber, heliotrope, musk, benzoin

A refined fragrance from Paris designer Jean-Louis Scherrer, Scherrer 2 is the fragrant equivalent of a silky Scherrer gown. An aldehydic top note is accented with soft fruits, while the radiant floral bouquet reverberates with subtle woods and amber. An understated feminine fragrance, ideal for exquisite afternoons of business or pleasure, and stunning evenings of mink and more.

Scherrer was a ballet student at the Paris Conservatory when an accident forced a career change. The rest is history. Scherrer honed his natural talent under the stellar tutelage of Christian Dior and Yves Saint Laurent. His first salon on the rue du Faubourg Saint-Honoré drew a titled clientele, from Empress Farah Diba to Baroness Thyssen and Princess Faisal.

Scherrer 2 is the successor to the original Scherrer fragrance.

Introduced   1986
Price   *Mid-range*

SECRET OF VENUS

Scent Type
  Floral - Oriental
Composition
  Notes: A Secret!

The French couture House of Weil introduced Secret of Venus at the end of World War II. It is an unusually rich, oil-based scent, simply packaged in an understated bottle accented with black and gold hues. Secret of Venus is best in cool weather, as it lasts and lasts.

What fun we had with this fragrance! When we asked the company what essences the fragrance contained, we were told that it had been ages since anyone had been able to locate that information, and the only folks who knew were the guardians of the formula, the laboratory chemists. And do they ever guard it...zealously! Never could get a straight reply, and even the industry tome from Haarmann & Reimer, *Fragrance Guide: Feminine Notes Masculine Notes,* couldn't shed light on the mystery, so the company suggested we put our team of expert noses to work on the problem. No guarantees, but here's what they sniffed: The top note is redolent of lavender, thyme and bergamot, while the heart of the fragrance suggests tuberose, jasmine, magnolia and rose. The symphony closes with musk, vanilla and wooded notes of sandalwood and patchouli, followed by a strong powdery finish. Actual ingredients, however, will remain the Secret of Venus...and its chemists.

Introduced   1945
Price   *Mid-range*

SENSO

Scent Type
  Floral - Fruity
Composition
  Top Notes: *Grapefruit, bergamot*
  Heart Notes: *Orange blossom, rose, jasmine*
  Base Notes: *Peppery carnation, sweet rose, jasmine*

The newest fragrance from Emanuel Ungaro, Senso is described as "the little sister of Diva," his first fragrance. Decidedly fruity, Senso is a light-spirited composition, an energetic scent aimed at a younger consumer. Nice for casual living and warm weather promenades.

The packaging was personally designed by Ungaro. The bottle is draped in magenta pink and crowned with a cobalt blue stopper that he says is "like a sapphire on a tiara." A vivid yellow polka-dot scarf is wrapped around the neck to complete the glorious presentation.

For the launch, Parfums Ungaro donated a portion of profits to the Make-A-Wish Foundation. The foundation has granted more than 14,000 wishes for children with terminal or life-threatening medical conditions. Ungaro designed a launch T-shirt bearing a French stamp with the words "1993 Wish."

Introduced   1993
Price   *Mid-range*

SHALIMAR

Scent Type
    Oriental
Composition
    Top Notes: *Bergamot, lemon, hesperides*
    Heart Notes: *Jasmine, iris, rose, patchouli, vetiver*
    Base Notes: *Vanilla, incense, opopanax, sandalwood, musk, civet, ambergris, leather*

Famous Patrons
    Meryl Streep
    Dionne Warwick
    Actress Josette Banzet

Shalimar is an intoxicating, yet subtly sensuous blend that has endured for more than sixty-five years. With a long-lasting base of spices and aromatic woods, it became the archetype for Oriental blends. A highly distinctive and dramatic fragrance, it was designed for the woman who is sensual, sophisticated and uninhibited...another grand entrance-making perfume from Guerlain.

A 1925 composition, Shalimar is reflective of its period, of a cosmopolitan Paris in the midst of celebration after World War I, of the Roaring Twenties, of exhilaration and new life. This attitude is mirrored in the zesty citrus top notes. Heady florals flow into a spicy drydown that is particularly rich in vanilla, incense and sandalwood.

In creating Shalimar, Jacques Guerlain was inspired by a love story told to him by a Maharajah visiting Paris. The Guerlain company shared the story with us:

More than 300 years ago, Shah Jahan succeeded to the throne of his father, Jahangir, and became the third Mogul Emperor of India.

Jahan loved only one woman. Her name was Mumtaz Mahal.

Some say he loved her unto madness, that she was not his wife but his fever.

*Victories, empires and riches were dust
as compared to her...in his eyes, she alone
was the balm that made life bearable.*

*When she died, Jahan's hair turned
white. He would burst into tears at the
mention of her name. In her memory,
he built one of the world's greatest
wonders—the Taj Mahal at Agra.*

*But the Taj Mahal is only an empty
monument. While Mumtaz was alive,
Jahan created a series of gardens for her
at Lahore, gardens the like of which had
never been seen before. He called them
the gardens of Shalimar, the Sanskrit
word meaning "abode of love."*

*From every corner of the Earth, the most
fragrant and delicate blossoms were
brought. Deep pools were built with
crystal fountains and terraces paved in
marble. The rarest birds were summoned
to sing here and lanterns were hung to
rival the stars. In the gardens of
Shalimar the lovers were truly happy,
and Mumtaz bore fourteen children
to her beloved Jahan.*

Jacques Guerlain decided that the perfume
should be called Shalimar, not Taj Mahal, because,
you see, Taj Mahal marks the end of the story,
and this love story can never end.... The flacon
was designed by Raymond Guerlain and is also
a reminder of the fountains in the gardens of
Shalimar. The ornamental stopper in sapphire
blue evokes the flow of the fountains' water.

Voluptuous and enveloping, Shalimar is a
fragrance of eternal romance. Look for Shalimar
bath and body products to extend your fragrance.

Introduced   1925
Price   High range

SMALTO DONNA

Scent Type
    Floral - Fruity
Composition
    Top Notes: *Living blue iris,
    Sicilian mandarin, living pear, tagetes*
    Heart Notes: *Tuberose, clove,
    orange blossom, ylang-ylang*
    Base Notes: *Indian sandalwood,
    opopanax, honey*

Designer Francesco Smalto launched Smalto
Donna in Cannes, France, to celebrate his entry
into the women's *prêt-à-porter* arena in 1993.

Smalto's designs served as inspiration
for the fragrance. Sparse elegance, clean and
uncomplicated are the watchwords. Fresh fruits
are blended with a dominant note of living blue
iris, while florals and spices are woven into a soft
base of sandalwood and honey. Easy to wear,
from office to home to casual nights.

Smalto Donna comes in bath and body
products, too. Look for it in coral cartons.

Introduced   1993
Price   Mid-range

SOCIETY BY BURBERRYS

Scent Type
Floral

Composition
Top Notes: *Black currant bud, tuberose, orange blossom, osmanthus, bergamot, hyacinth, greens*
Heart Notes: *Jasmine, mimosa, iris, ylang-ylang, gardenia, rose, orchid, lily of the valley*
Base Notes: *Patchouli, oakmoss, myrrh, frankincense, cedarwood, amber, musk, vanilla*

Society is a scent introduced by British-based Burberrys. Upon its debut, it was honored with a prestigious industry award, the FiFi. Society is an elegant, sophisticated floral fragrance, eminently suitable for a society lady.

The fragrance begins with a floral accord enhanced by greens and bergamot for a fresh lift. A rich blend of exotic florals and soothing, powdery woods complete the composition.

Society comes in sculpted glass containers, topped with ruby-colored caps embellished with the Burberry logo, a silver porsum knight. Try the bath and body line for a real treat.

Introduced   1991
Price   High range

SONIA RYKIEL

Scent Type
Semi-Oriental

Composition
Top Notes: *Mandarin, ylang-ylang, Hinoki wood, passion flower*
Heart Notes: *Jasmine, May rose, lily of the valley, iris, sandalwood, patchouli*
Base Notes: *Vanilla, amber, tonka bean, benzoin*

Before you slip into your Sonia Rykiel knitwear, spritz on her signature fragrance. It is designed to be just as comfortable and sensual as the easy, elegant fashions for which she is known. For the introduction, Rykiel displayed an enormous poster above her Paris headquarters featuring a woman lifting her sweater with the phrase, "Under my sweater, the perfume." We understand it caused a stir among passer-bys, resulting in honks, whistles and slowed traffic.

The semi-Oriental fragrance is a subtle, refined blend meant more for the personal enjoyment of the wearer than for others. It is equally appropriate for private moments or professional career wear, whenever an under-stated fragrance is desired.

Introduced   1993 (Europe)
Price   Mid-range

SPELLBOUND

Scent Type
Floral - Ambery

Composition
Top Notes: Fruits, rosewood, coriander, orange blossom, pimento
Heart Notes: Rose, jasmine, tuberose, carnation, lily of the valley, carnation, heliotrope
Base Notes: Vanilla, amber, cedarwood, benzoin, musk, civet, opopanax

Estée Lauder brings us yet another fragrance destined to be a classic. Spellbound casts a potent spell with spices, rare flowers and exotic woods woven into a sophisticated ambery blend with Oriental accents. A clove-like aroma adds impact to the dramatic, feminine statement.

The magical scent is encased in a classic glass bottle topped with a sleek brass ornament.

Introduced   1991
Price   High range

SPOILED

Scent Type
Floral

Composition
Top Notes: Mandarin, bergamot, greens, herbs, coriander, tagetes
Heart Notes: Jasmine, orange blossom, rose, ylang-ylang, lily of the valley
Base Notes: Amber, musk, spices

Theodore of Beverly Hills brings us Spoiled, a scent that scintillates with fruity green top notes and voluptuous florals. Amber and musk are massaged into a backdrop that reeks of a world of Lagondas, trysts and trust funds.

One would expect a fragrance of this name from Beverly Hills. Ah, that this Beverly Hills author were only that spoiled! But we're working on it....

Introduced   1987
Price   High range

SUBLIME

Scent Type
Floral

Composition
Top and Heart Notes: Pure flowers, jasmine, rose
Base Notes: Amber, musk

Famous Patrons
Actress Alessandra Martines

Sublime is a superb fragrance from the French firm of Jean Patou that brought the world the scent of Joy. The company says Sublime is "an instant of sheer happiness, of pure delight." It was designed for the modern woman, radiant and sensual, tender and opulent, who is "equally at ease frolicking in a whimsical garden as she is basking in the Parisian sunlight on the banks of the Seine."

Famed French film maker Claude Lelouch provided the artistry evident in the photography of Italian actress Alessandra Martines, the sublime woman used in the print advertising. The flacon carries out the sublime vision—curved to fit a woman's hand, endowed with a gold-colored stopper in the shape of a flower bud...all in shades of brilliant amber and gold.

The scent is rife with pure floral essences, warmed by golden amber and sensual musk tones. Sublime is an opulent floral bouquet in the rich tradition of Jean Patou, understated for the nineties.

Introduced   1993
Price   High range

SUNFLOWERS

Scent Type
    Floral - Fruity
Composition
    Top Notes: Bergamot, melon, peach
    Heart Notes: Jasmine, cyclamen, tea rose, osmanthus
    Base Notes: Sandalwood, musk, moss

Famous Patrons
    Model Vendela

Sunflowers is a brisk fruity floral from Elizabeth Arden, ideal for spa lovers. Arden calls it a "prestige fragrance without the prestige pricing." Created in response to the nineties woman's attraction to all things natural, Sunflowers is light enough to be worn by women of any age, and is perfect for casual, outdoor and warm weather use. We love it on the tennis court, or for a leisurely bicycle ride through the country.

Sunflowers is presented in a package with a sunflower cut-out, and the fragrance itself is in a simple clear glass bottle imprinted with the name in bright white and yellow. The fragrance is available in a light eau de toilette only, but can be layered with the perfumed body lotion and the bath/shower gelee for longer-lasting Sunflowers.

A romantic note appears on the side of the box: "And the sun was shining when he held me and I felt a deep flowering of pleasure. All at once. Like a sunflower. Opening up." We just love the return to romance.

Introduced   1993
Price   Mid range

SUNG, ALFRED SUNG

Scent Type
    Floral - Green
Composition
    Top Notes: Orange, ylang-ylang, mandarin, bergamot, galbanum, lemon, hyacinth
    Heart Notes: Osmanthus, genet, jasmine, iris, lily of the valley
    Base Notes: Vanilla, orange blossom, sandalwood, ambrette, vetiver

Sung is the first fragrance from international designer Alfred Sung. He states, "My perfume is an extension of my designs, an evolution, an intimate expression of a woman's wants and desires." First launched in Canada in 1986 and followed by a 1988 U.S. introduction, Sung enjoyed immediate success.

The signature white floral fragrance features sparkling fresh citrus blended with green notes and white flowers, set against a refined backdrop of woods and spices. Fresh and light, it is a classic fragrance that can be worn with equal ease on the shores of Palm Beach, to Manhattan galas or on Swiss slopes.

The feminine, sophisticated floral is encased in a classic Pierre Dinand bottle of clean, uncomplicated, symmetrical lines.

To experience the ultimate luxury, pamper your entire body with the Sung Essential Bath and Body Collection.

Introduced 1986
Price High range

SWEET COURRÈGES

Scent Type
Floral - Fruity
Composition
Top Notes: Watermelon, grapefruit, passion fruit
Heart Notes: White florals, white cyclamen, lilac, freesia
Base Notes: Cedarwood, vanilla, sandalwood

The fourth women's fragrance from André Courrèges is Sweet Courrèges. As the name suggests, the sweet concoction is a blend of tropical fruits and light white flowers against a soft wooded background. The tender scent is pretty for hot days, close quarters and youthful innocence.

Appropriately colored in pale pink, the wrapping is based on a pink and white ruffled dress from the Courrèges collection. A fitting garment for the feminine fragrance.

Introduced 1993 (Europe)
1994 (United States)
Price Mid-range

TAMANGO

Scent Type
Floral - Aldehyde
Composition
Top Notes: Aldehydes, hyacinth, iris, wild orchid
Heart Notes: Rose, lily of the valley, jasmine
Base Notes: Sandalwood, oakmoss, vetiver, musk

Tamango is an exotic floral symphony with a dominant note of wild orchids, lifted by ethereal aldehydic top notes and soothed with soft sandalwood and oakmoss. Feminine, rich, refined. The classic fragrance from Léonard Parfums is sealed in a Serge Mansau-designed bottle and tucked in a black package, kissed with a symbolic wild orchid.

Introduced   1977
Price   Mid-range

TATIANA

Scent Type
  Floral
Composition
  Top Notes: *Orange blossom, bergamot, greens*
  Heart Notes: *Jasmine, jonquil, tuberose, narcissus, rose*
  Base Notes: *Sandalwood, musk, civet*

Tatiana is a luminous floral bouquet created by designer Diane Von Furstenberg. It is a sweet, diffusive floral with refreshing underlying green notes. A strong jasmine floral complex develops through the middle drying to a powdery floral base.

Inspired by her young daughter Tatiana, Von Furstenberg decided to name her first fragrance after her. She wanted a scent you could inhale the way you would fresh flowers. She succeeded in developing this wonderful floral that truly smelled good. Tatiana, the fragrance, was created for a woman to love and a man to remember. Tatiana, now a young woman herself; women still love it and men still remember it.

Tatiana was one of Von Furstenberg's many creations. We remember the sexy Diane Von Furstenberg wrap dress that everyone could wear—it slipped on quickly and took us almost everywhere. A trip to Bali resulted in the 1981 launch of her woman's fragrance, Volcan d'Amour,

an exotic floral, along with a new color palette for her already successful cosmetic line, The Color Authority. She has also designed successful lines of accessories, sportswear and home furnishings.

Look for Diane Von Furstenberg's beautiful books on home decor, *Beds* and *The Bath*. She can also be seen on QVC with her *Silk Assets* line of sportswear and *Surroundings*, scents for yourself and your environment.

Introduced   1975
Relaunched   1994
Price   Mid-range

TEATRO ALLA SCALA

Scent Type
  Oriental - Spicy
Composition
  Top Notes: *Coriander, bergamot, aldehydes, fruits*
  Heart Notes: *Rose, jasmine, ylang-ylang, carnation, tuberose, geranium, orris, beeswax*
  Base Notes: *Patchouli, vetiver, civet, moss, musk, cistus, benzoin*

Teatro alla Scala is a beautifully balanced Oriental fragrance from Krizia with a soft backdrop of woods and subtle spices. Florals, fruits and aldehydic notes are harmonized into an easy-to-wear Oriental blend that is versatile enough to span a variety of seasons and events.

Teatro alla Scala borrows its name from the famous Italian theater. The drama is carried out through the flacon amidst heated swirls of amber and orange. To really shine, slip it into your Judith L. dazzle bag for opening night at a London theater.

Introduced   1986
Price   High range

TENDRE POISON

Scent Type
  Floral - Fresh
Composition
  Top Notes: *Galbanum, mandarin*
  Heart Notes: *Freesia, orange, honey*
  Base Notes: *Vanilla, sandalwood*

Christian Dior's original Poison has gone green with its fresh counterpart, Tendre Poison. The fragrance is positioned to appeal to a younger market, or those who want a change from the heady, erotic aroma of the original Poison.

Lightness is achieved with top notes of green galbanum and smooth fruity mandarin, before moving to an ethereal heart led by freesia. The drydown is soft yet tenacious, with the sweetness of sandalwood and vanilla.

Tendre Poison shares packaging and bottles with its more mature sibling, though in green, of course. With Tendre Poison, Christian Dior proves the old adage false: The grass is not always greener on the other side.

Introduced   1994
Price   High range

360 PERRY ELLIS

Scent Type
  Floral
Composition
  Top Notes: *Melon, tangerine, osmanthus, lily, cool blue rose*
  Heart Notes: *Lily of the valley, lavender, water lily, sage*
  Base Notes: *Sandalwood, vanilla, vetiver, amber, musk*

The latest fragrance from the Perry Ellis fragrance team is 360, a musky floral blend that re-creates the late American designer's energetic outlook.

Packaging was a collaboration between Perry Ellis design teams and bottle designer Marc Rosen. A silvery ring encircles the round package that the company says is meant to suggest "a crystal ball, a full moon, a perfect pearl." The eau de toilette is held in a sleek cylinder topped with another 360 sphere.

The 1993 launch party was appropriately held at Ellis Island. Festivities revolved around a picnic, fireworks and entertainment by the American Boys Choir of Princeton.

Introduced   1993
Price   High range

TIANNE

Scent Type
  Oriental - Spicy

Composition
    Top Notes: *Florals*
    Heart Notes: *Florals, spices*
    Base Notes: *Woods, spices*

Famous Patrons
    Mamie Eisenhower

Tianne is a spice blend that was launched in the 1950s by Nettie Rosenstein, whose fashion line is no longer in existence. Tianne is one of the surviving trio of her women's fragrances.

Discernable fragrance notes suggest a floral spice blend of coriander, nutmeg, cinnamon, ginger, bay leaf, lavender and carnation. The fragrance lingers with a woody, powdery aroma.

Look for Tianne at select stores, packaged in colors of blue and gold with a signature bow.

Introduced   1950s
Price   Mid-range

TIFFANY

Scent Type
    Floral - Ambery

Composition
    Top Notes: *Indian jasmine, Damascena rose, ylang-ylang, mandarin, orange blossom, Italian mandarin*
    Heart Notes: *Florentine iris, lily of the valley, black currant bud, violet leaves*
    Base Notes: *Sandalwood, amber, vanilla, vetiver*

Famous Patrons
    Fashion designer Vera Wang

Tiffany is the signature fragrance from the world-renowned retailer of fine jewelry, timepieces, accessories and tableware. An effusive bouquet of 150 floral notes, the Tiffany fragrance was created in 1987 in honor of the 150th anniversary of Tiffany & Company.

The fragrance begins with fruity top notes that give way to a refined semi-Oriental arrangement of florals, aromatic woods and sweet vanilla. A sophisticated fragrance, Tiffany is equally suitable for the office and romantic dinners.

Tiffany Design Director John Loring and famed bottle designer Pierre Dinand created the elegant Art Deco bottle that houses the subtle, distinctive perfume. It is packaged, of course, in Tiffany's signature color of robin's-egg blue. The fragrance and body care line are available at Tiffany stores, as well as fine department stores.

Tiffany has been a supporter of the Susan G. Komen Breast Cancer Foundation since 1986. Tiffany designed a scarf and accessories in honor of the Foundation and donated a percentage of profit from each sale. For 1993, the company set a goal of donating $100,000. The Foundation was started in 1982 by Nancy Brinker in honor of her sister who died at age 36 of breast cancer. The Komen Foundation offers information on breast cancer prevention at 1-800-I'M-AWARE.

Introduced   1987
Price   High range

TRÉSOR

Scent Type
Floral Semi-Oriental

Composition
Top Notes: *Rose, apricot blossom, lilac, peach*
Heart Notes: *Iris, heliotrope, lily of the valley, jasmine*
Base Notes: *Amber, sandalwood, musk, vanilla*

Famous Patrons
Isabella Rossellini

From the French word for "treasure," Lancôme's Trésor was designed as a round fragrance, where the head, heart and drydown notes blend together. Trésor is laden with fruits, florals and long-lasting Oriental base notes. It is a saucy daytime fragrance, yet versatile enough to dress up for evening. Fresh, spirited and innocent. We love it in warm weather, especially après spa.

The clear glass bottle is shaped like an inverted pyramid, designed by Areca to represent the glowing radiance of a woman in full bloom. Reflective of its fresh peach and apricot essences, the fragrance is presented in peach and salmon floral packaging. It is, indeed, a treasure.

Introduced   1991
Price   High range

TRIBÙ

Scent Type
Floral - Fruity

Composition
Top Notes: *African tagetes, Italian violet leaves, Belgian black currant bud, Italian mandarin*
Heart Notes: *Bulgarian rose, Moroccan geranium, Indonesian ylang-ylang, Egyptian chamomile, Moroccan jasmine*
Base Notes: *Indian sandalwood, Haitian vetiver, Yugoslavian oakmoss, Thai benzoin*

Famous Patrons
Frank Sinatra and family
Sonia Braga
Roberta Flack

From the United Colors of Benetton comes Tribù, described by the company as a "fragrance and bath ritual collection that celebrates the tribal roots of all human beings, transcending time, cultures and ethnicity."

Sunny top notes register green apple, peach and mandarin orange, followed by delicate flowers embedded in sweet lasting notes of sandalwood and ambery benzoin.

Made from healthy all-natural ingredients from around the world, Tribù is housed in an amber and red flacon designed by Tamotsu Yagi, and its packaging is made from recycled paper. The elongated bottle is part of the permanent collection at the San Francisco Museum of Modern Art. Yagi drew inspiration from an egg, one of the most primitive design forms, and a test tube, a symbol of the modern age. The ad campaign from avant-garde award-winning photographer Oliviero Toscani depicts real people, not models, practicing ancient and modern tribal rituals, many culled from the archives of National Geographic.

All this and Frank Sinatra, too. His 1938 classic love song, "I'll Be Seeing You," is the theme song. Benetton believes that, like Tribù, Frank Sinatra's song and style span diverse cultures and generations.

Introduced   1992
Price   Mid-range

TUBÉREUSE

Scent Type
Floral
Composition
Notes: *Grasse tuberose*

Tuberose is an extraordinarily fragrant white flower, and perhaps the finest tuberose in the world is found in Grasse, France. Creator Annick Goutal describes Tubéreuse as "a keynote of irresistible fascination. A scent for the woman with mysterious powers of seduction." Tubéreuse is a heady, beguiling fragrance.

In the language of flowers, tuberose represents dangerous pleasures. Try this and report back to us—we have a steamy novel in the works and can use more material!

Introduced   1986
Price   Top range

TUSCANY PER DONNA

Scent Type
Floral - Oriental
Composition
Top Notes: *Mandarin, grapefruit, bergamot, rose, hyacinth, lily of the valley, herbs*
Heart Notes: *Jasmine, honeysuckle, ylang-ylang, orange blossom, violet, carnation*
Base Notes: *Sandalwood, vanilla, amber, musk*

Tuscany Per Donna is a fragrance from Aramis, an Estée Lauder company. It was introduced to complement Aramis' successful men's fragrance, Tuscany. The subtle scent takes its inspiration from the tranquillity of the Tuscan countryside and the Italian Renaissance woman.

Tuscany Per Donna opens with a shimmering tumble of florals, citrus fruits and herbs. The body unfolds with rich florals, then softens into a background accord of fragrant woods and sweet spices; like Italy in the spring.

Tuscany Per Donna is housed in handsome copper and amber leaded glass flacons, and tapestry print packages.

Introduced   1993
Price   Mid-range

273 FOR WOMEN

Scent Type
Floral

Composition
Top Notes: Gardenia, tuberose, jasmine, peach, plum
Heart Notes: Peach, apricot, ylang-ylang, orris
Base Notes: Sandalwood, vetiver, amber, spices, cedarwood

Fred Hayman created 273 in the finest tradition to reflect the desires of his elegant international clientele. 273 takes its name, of course, from the address of Fred Hayman's store at 273 North Rodeo Drive, Beverly Hills. The Swiss-born Hayman relied on the collective critiques of his store's clientele in developing this scent, which was nearly two years in the making. He created a VIP Fragrance Panel of prominent women to contribute their expertise and opinions.

The fragrance is a velvety floral of more than 250 ingredients—classic rich florals, exotic spices, smoldering amber and earthy woods. Elegant and easy to wear, 273 is a smooth harmony.

The fragrance is housed in a pyramid-shaped bottle, with a stopper encircled by a 24-karat gold band. The entire vibrant yellow presentation captures the sophisticated spirit and fun of sunny Southern California.

Introduced	1989
Price	Mid-range

UN JOUR

Scent Type
Floral

Composition
Top Notes: Sicilian mandarin, black currant bud, peach, lemon, pineapple, greens
Heart Notes: Jasmine, white royal lily, magnolia, ylang-ylang, hyacinth
Base Notes: Virginia cedarwood, West Indian rosewood, oakmoss, musk, sandalwood

Un Jour is a fruity floral from couturier Charles Jourdan. The radiant light floral is accented with fresh green notes and underscored with mild, powdery woods.

Un Jour, meaning "a day" in French, is like an armful of wildflowers on a sunny summer day. A versatile daytime fragrance.

Introduced	1978
Price	Mid-range

UNGARO

Scent Type
Oriental - Ambery

Composition
Top Notes: Neroli, jasmine, orange blossom, rose essence
Heart Notes: Turkish rose, Florentine iris
Base Notes: Tonka bean, cardamom, sandalwood, amber

Following his successful Diva, Emanuel Ungaro introduced his signature fragrance—an Oriental blend with warm ambery base notes. Enthralling and exotic, just like Ungaro fashion.

The bottle mimics Ungaro's signature fashion drape, like a one-shouldered dress or a flowing Greek robe. The flacon is a deep midnight blue, topped with an emerald-colored faceted glass stopper, accented with a fuchsia ribbon at the neck. It is a true work of art from Jacques Helleu for Ungaro.

Introduced   1991
Price   Top range

V'E VERSACE

Scent Type
  Chypre - Floral
Composition
  Top Notes: Bergamot, lily of the valley, Bulgarian rose, jasmine, ylang-ylang, lily
  Heart Notes: Orange blossom, iris
  Base Notes: Balsamic wood, incense, amber, sandalwood, oakmoss

Famous Patrons
  Cher
  Elizabeth Taylor
  Tina Turner
  Also bought by Sting, Sylvester Stallone, Bruce Springsteen and Elton John for their women

Milano fashion daredevil Gianni Versace says: "I don't care for half-measures. I believe in making clear-cut choices." Indeed he does. Versace is the designer who turned chain metal mail into evening wear. An extremist in his work, he is a risk taker who has ushered in striking styles for the young couture group.

Now he expresses himself through his latest fragrance, V'E Versace. The scent derives its name from a shorthand, simpatico signature, with a Mediterranean slant. A sensual fragrance, it resonates with vivid, white florals embedded in provocative base notes of incense and balsamic woods.

The bottle is described as "a cube which is not a cube," a modern, futuristic creation showcasing trademark Versace asymmetry. His own solid crystal inkwell served as inspiration. He also produced a limited edition Baccarat crystal flacon. Only 250 were made, each requiring a week of patient, skilled artistry. A lofty purchase, priced at about $3,500.

V'E Versace is also available in body and bath products, from shower gels to soaps and lotion. They complete the expression of V'E. As the designer explains: "Human beings need room to express themselves, that is why we should have the courage to declare *Liberta de Profumo!* This expression allows us to break away from the roles and regulations that we often set for ourselves."

Introduced   1993
Price   High range

VAN CLEEF & ARPELS

Scent Type
Floral - Oriental

Composition
Top Notes: Neroli, bergamot, raspberry, galbanum
Heart Notes: Rose, jasmine, orange blossom
Base Notes: Cedarwood, vanilla, musk, tonka bean

The 1993 signature fragrance from Van Cleef & Arpels jewelers is a renewed commitment to the parfum extract fragrance strength. Available only in the longer-lasting perfume and eau de parfum strengths, the floral Oriental blend is also surprisingly well-priced. How did they manage that feat? By simplifying packaging and using only one bottle type. Smart!

Breezy top notes of fruits and greens enliven a rich floral heart, while warm Oriental base notes linger with subtle opulence. A feminine, refined fragrance with a superb pedigree.

Look for the scent in an asymmetric gem-faceted flacon by designer Serge Mansau. Jewel tones of ivory, gold and lapis blue clothe the precious fragrance.

Introduced 1993 (Europe)
1994 (United States)
Price Mid-range

VANDERBILT

Scent Type
Floral - Oriental

Composition
Top Notes: Orange blossom, apricot, bergamot, greens, mandarin, coriander, basil
Heart Notes: Rose, jasmine, jonquil, mimosa absolute
Base Notes: Musk, amber, moss, incense, vanilla

Vanderbilt was created in honor of Gloria Vanderbilt and her legendary family name, the very mention of which conjures up images of luxury and grandeur from a bygone era.

The romantic fragrance is a light floral Oriental. Herbs, fruits and spices introduce the lush floral heart, where dominant essences of rose and jasmine reside. The background is a harmony of warm Oriental notes, powdery, rich and sweet. Vanderbilt is a charming fragrance that is fitting for young and old.

The perfume is housed in a bottle by Bernard Kotyuk. It bears the Vanderbilt signature and is crowned with a Lalique-style stopper, in which a graceful swan is carved. The swan logo is carried throughout other packaging, symbolizing grace and elegance.

A new addition to the fragrance, body and bath line is Satin Parfum, an alcohol-free perfume that hydrates and softens the skin. The Vanderbilt fragrance is available in a wide array of attractively priced products.

Introduced 1982
Price Mid-range

VENDETTA

Scent Type
  Floral - Oriental
Composition
  Top Notes: Water lily, hyacinth,
  orange blossom
  Heart Notes: Rose, jasmine, ylang-ylang,
  daffodil, marigold
  Base Notes: Musk, sandalwood, patchouli

From Italian couturier Valentino comes
Vendetta, a dramatic floral Oriental with fresh
top notes. The simmering, sensuous scent
embodies his passion for elegant, timeless and
fiery creations.

Valentino has dressed some of the
legendary women of our time, including Jackie
Onassis, Sophia Loren, Princess Diana and
Elizabeth Taylor.

The strong floral bouquet is encased in
a stunning Serge Mansau-designed bottle,
evocative of rippling draped fabric or a plissé
fan, and packaged in Valentino red and zebra-
patterned black. The marketing gurus borrow
a line from Bizet's "Carmen" to describe the
scent: "If you don't love me, I love you, and if
I love you, be careful." Hot, hot, hot.

Introduced	1993
Price	Top range

VENEZIA

Scent Type
  Floral - Oriental
Composition
  Top Notes: Wong-shi blossom,
  Indian mango, black currant bud, rose,
  geranium, prune, osmanthus
  Heart Notes: Jasmine, iris, ylang-ylang,
  cedarwood, ambergris
  Base Notes: Vanilla, civet, sandalwood,
  musk, tonka bean

Famous Patrons
  Ann-Margret

For her second scent, Venezia, Italian
fashion designer Laura Biagiotti took inspiration
from the ancient city of canals, magical Venice.
She describes Venezia as "Aromas from the
Orient and the Occident merged into a perfume
of infinite richness."

The initial prevailing notes of Venezia are
the essence of fruits mingled with wong-shi
blossom, a rare gardenia-like flower that Marco
Polo brought to Venice from the Orient. The
flower was admired by Medieval Venetians.
Italian poets called it *"l'eliser d'amore,"* the elixir
of love. Captivated by the rare essence, Laura
Biagiotti based her fragrance upon it as a tribute
to the irresistible city of Venice. As the
fragrance develops on the skin, a bouquet of
rich florals and woods emerges, giving way to
a sensual balsamic Oriental base.

The spicy, seductive scent is encased in
a Venetian-style glass bottle inspired by the

Harlequin, the most important figure in Venetian carnivals. Fine gold shavings float in the perfume, while the cap is a recreation of the campanile of San Giorgio Maggiore. The gilded packaging features a winged lion, the symbol of Venice, in Harlequin colors of gold and red. The Venezia packaging and fragrance are splendid works of modern Italian art.

Introduced 1992
Price Top range

VENT VERT

Scent Type
  Floral - Green
Composition
  Top Notes: *Greens, orange blossom, lemon, lime, basil*
  Heart Notes: *Rose, galbanum, lily of the valley, freesia, hyacinth, tagetes, ylang-ylang, violet*
  Base Notes: *Oakmoss, sandalwood, sage, iris, amber, musk*

Vent Vert is a green floral from Paris couturier Pierre Balmain. The company describes the vibrant sharp fragrance, saying it is "an exhilarating fragrance, evocative of nature in spring: subtle scents of mown grass, fresh flower buds and blossoms gracefully mingling in a light breeze." Green and mossy notes are woven throughout the composition. In fact, Vent Vert is French for "green breeze."

The green theme is carried out in crisp mint green packaging. When you want a light, clean fragrance for daytime or professional wear, try Vent Vert, a fresh understated floral.

Introduced 1947
Price High range

VERSUS FOR WOMEN

Scent Type
  Floral - Fruity
Composition
  Top Notes: *Raspberry, plum, black currant bud*
  Heart Notes: *Tuberose, boronia, sandalwood*
  Base Notes: *Iris, amber, musk*

Famous Patrons
  Model Carla Bruni

Maverick Gianni Versace formulated Versus to complement his expressive, avant-garde fashions. He heads a family-run empire that caters to dynamic youth, offering his body-hugging flamboyant styles. The fruity floral fragrance is a youthful, defiant, sensual scent, positioned to appeal to the MTV generation.

Versace describes the Versus woman as "electrifying, sensual and habitually unattainable." Supermodel Carla Bruni is the Versus woman, the woman who "creates her own rules and forges her own path." Bruni is featured in the advertising campaign, along with plenty of leather and a Harley motorcycle.

Versus was launched at Miami's ultra-trendy South Beach hotel, the Raleigh. Just so happens, Versace recently introduced his book of a similar name, *South Beach Stories*.

The ruby red bottles and lipstick-red cap are accented by a gold-colored collar and deep sculpted "V." Defiant and dramatic...pure Versace.

Introduced   *1992*
Price   *Mid-range*

VICKY TIEL

Scent Type
Floral
Composition
    Top Notes: *Oriental mandarin, Italian bergamot, lemon, neroli, greens*
    Heart Notes: *Jasmine, narcissus, lily of the valley, jonquil, rose, orchid, broom, ylang-ylang*
    Base Notes: *Indian sandalwood, tuberose, camellia, oakmoss, musk, amber, heliotrope, cedarwood*

Vicky Tiel is the namesake fragrance from exclusive couturier Vicky Tiel. Tangy essence of bergamot and mandarin introduce the ambrosial scent, which develops into a sophisticated blend of fragrant white flowers reputed to be aphrodisiacs. Lingering notes of sweet woods, mosses and florals complete the compelling, feminine scent. Certainly a head-turning fragrance.

The Vicky Tiel perfume is encased in a bottle of frosted aqua crystal, embellished with female silhouettes in skillfully carved relief. The stopper is signed by Vicky Tiel and holds a surprise—the application wand is a sculpted female figurine, ready to trail the exquisite fragrance from her toes. It is a fabulous creation, destined to be a collector's item.

Introduced   *1991*
Price   *Top range*

VIVID

Scent Type
Floral
Composition
    Top Notes: *Egyptian marigold, tangerine, bergamot, violet, freesia*
    Heart Notes: *Tiare flower, jasmine, peony, iris, lilies, Bulgarian rose*
    Base Notes: *Sandalwood, musk, vanilla, amber*

Liz Claiborne Cosmetics describes Vivid, as "exotic, romantic, feminine and sophisticated." The signature note is tiare flower, a blossom with a rare long-lasting essence. Vivid means "full of life," just like the woman for whom it was created. The fragrance begins with crisp and fruity top notes, followed by a rich floral heart. The lasting floral impression is warmed by sweet vanilla and amber, enhanced by musk and softened by sandalwood.

The Vivid perfume is contained in a weighted round flacon, while Vivid eau de toilette products are housed in curved tear-shaped silhouettes. The line includes a moisturizing body lotion, while bath products are scheduled for a Fall 1994 release. Ribboned accents and woven patterns are nods to the Liz Claiborne clothing heritage.

Introduced   1993
Price   High range

VOL DE NUIT

Scent Type
Oriental - Ambery Spicy
Composition
Top Notes: Orange, mandarin, lemon, bergamot, orange blossom
Heart Notes: Jonquil, aldehydes, galbanum
Base Notes: Vanilla, spices, oakmoss, sandalwood, orris, musk

Another timeless classic from Jacques Guerlain, Vol de Nuit is a spicy Oriental scent designed for the elusive, assertive woman, and is one of the most sophisticated scents from the House of Guerlain.

Vol de Nuit, French for "night flight," is presented in one of our favorite Guerlain flacons. The dramatic gold-colored amber bottle is molded with the shape of French Air Force wings. Indeed, Vol de Nuit was created in homage to the daring aviators of the 1920s, and was named after the Antoine de Saint-

Exupéry novel of the same name. Saint-Exupéry, also an avid aviator, was the author of many works, including *Le Petit Prince*.

The fragrance captures the essence of adventure, the spirit of exploration, the radiance of independence. It is an assertive scent of the thirties; ideal for the woman of the nineties.

Introduced   1933
Price   High range

VOLCAN D'AMOUR

Scent Type
Floral
Composition
Top Notes: Violet, orange blossom, tagetes, ylang-ylang
Heart Notes: Lily of the valley, jasmine, rose, tuberose
Base Notes: Moss, sandalwood, musk, patchouli, vetiver

Volcan D'Amour is a provocative creation by Diane Von Furstenberg, following on the success of her first fragrance, Tatiana. The exotic floral features an alluring violet top note surrounded by orris, mingling with precious woods of vetiver, sandalwood and patchouli, laced with fragrant mosses.

A trip to Bali served as inspiration for the passionate launch of Volcan D'Amour, or "volcano of love." It was there Von Furstenberg heard the legend of Vulcan, the god of fire, and Venus, the goddess of love, who married each other and resided on the volcano Mt. Etna, where the violets used in fragrance grow. The Bali trip inspired these poetic words:

> *Into my life you came,*
> *Bringing peace to my heart,*
> *Fire to my body,*
> *Love to my soul,*
> *In your eyes I see myself,*
> *Feeling, reaching, looking*
> *For perfect harmony.*
> *Diane Von Furstenberg, Bali 1980*

Volcan D'Amour is housed in an exquisite bottle by renowned bottle designer Dakota Jackson.

Introduced	*1981*
Relaunch planned	*1994-95*
Price	*High range*

VOLUPTÉ

Scent Type
    Floral - Oriental
Composition
    Top Notes: *Living mimosa, living freesia, living osmanthus, tagetes, mandarin, melon*
    Heart Notes: *Jasmine, heliotrope, ylang-ylang, carnation, lily of the valley*
    Base Notes: *Sandalwood, amber, patchouli, incense*

Famous Patrons
    Princess Margaret

Volupté, meaning "voluptuous," is an effervescent fragrance from Santo Domingo couturier Oscar de la Renta, distributed by Sanofi Beaute in North America.

Volupté is meant to represent "unequaled sensual appeal." A warm, exotic Oriental blend, it is highlighted with spirited touches of melon and mandarin for elegant, fresh, understated seduction. Living flower technology enabled de la Renta to faithfully reproduce the essence of live blooming flowers, including mimosa and freesia.

The fragrance garnered two 1993 FiFi Awards from The Fragrance Foundation for excellence: best women's fragrance in broad distribution and best women's fragrance package.

The seductive fragrance comes in an elegant bottle from designer Pierre Dinand; a graceful, fluid creation with gold- and emerald-colored accents. The special crystal edition is gorgeous, and holds a full ounce of the fragrance—a lovely treat for about $300.

Introduced	*1992*
Price	*High Range*

VÔTRE

Scent Type
Floral

Composition
Top Notes: *Hyacinth, mandarin, galbanum, cassie, spices, aldehydes*
Heart Notes: *French marigold, plum tree evernia, ylang-ylang, jasmine, rose, lily of the valley*
Base Notes: *Sandalwood, amber, cedarwood, musk, raspberry*

Couturier Charles Jourdan used more than 130 rare essential oils to form Vôtre. Fruits, spices and greens create a sassy top note, while radiant florals and mild woods smooth the composition.

Vôtre means "yours" in French. It can be yours in any language.

Introduced   1979
Price   *Mid-range*

WEIL DE WEIL

Scent Type
Floral - Green

Composition
Top Notes: *Tangerine, neroli, greens, galbanum, hyacinth*
Heart Notes: *Lily of the valley, honeysuckle, ylang-ylang, acacia farnesiana, May rose, narcissus*
Base Notes: *Sandalwood, vetiver, civet, musk, oakmoss*

The classic Weil de Weil begins with saucy citrus and lively green notes, blended with a symphony of fragrant white flowers, and couched in a bed of sandalwood warmed by woody vetiver and soft, erotic musk.

Weil de Weil...a green floral bouquet well worth the experiment.

Introduced   1971
Price   *Mid-range*

WHITE DIAMONDS

Scent Type
Floral

Composition
Top Notes: *Italian neroli, living Amazon lily, aldehydes*
Heart Notes: *Egyptian tuberose, Turkish rose, Italian orris, living narcissus, living jasmine*
Base Notes: *Italian sandalwood, patchouli, amber, oakmoss*

As with her first fragrance, Passion, Elizabeth Taylor again proves able to translate her extraordinary sense of style to a seemingly innate sense of scent. She calls White Diamonds "the fragrance that dreams are made of."

A dazzling combination of floral essences and sparkling aldehydes are blended to create a floral fragrance that is delicate yet tenacious, with a subtle Oriental drydown. White Diamonds is a sophisticated floral bouquet, versatile enough to be worn for casually elegant days and lavish evenings...anytime you'd wear diamonds.

White Diamonds inhabits a brilliant bottle. Like those of the gemstone trio of Diamonds and Emeralds, Diamonds and Rubies, and Diamonds and Sapphires, the White Diamonds eau de parfum columnar spray bottles are adorned with a generous band of shimmering *faux* and pavé crystal stones, while the oval-shaped perfume bottle is dressed with a glittering rhinestone bow. We love it; diamonds may be a woman's best friend, but *faux* diamonds cost much less to insure.

The packaging has received numerous accolades from industry peers, notably a 1992 FiFi Award from The Fragrance Foundation, the fragrance industry equivalent of an Oscar. Taylor was graciously on hand to accept the honor.

Introduced   1991
Price   *High range*

WHITE LINEN

Scent Type
  Floral - Aldehyde
Composition
  Top Notes: *Aldehydes, peach, citrus oils*
  Heart Notes: *Jasmine, lilac, rose, hyacinth, lily of the valley, orchid, ylang-ylang*
  Base Notes: *Amber, cedarwood, sandalwood, honey, benzoin, tonka bean*

Estée Lauder was searching for the fragrance embodiment of white linen, the look and the meaning—clean, crisp and classic. Always right. She achieved this in the development of White Linen, the fragrance.

The bouquet of delicate florals is introduced by airy top notes of shimmering aldehydes. The scent lingers on base notes of warm woods and spices to create an aura of understated elegance. Romantic and gentle, White Linen is a feminine scent with a polished demeanor. It is ideal for warm weather and subtle daytime wear...anytime you'd slip into pressed white linen.

Introduced   1978
Price   *High range*

WHITE SHOULDERS

Scent Type
  Floral
Composition
  Top Notes: *Neroli, tuberose, aldehydes*
  Heart Notes: *Gardenia, jasmine, orris, lily of the valley, rose, lilac*
  Base Notes: *Sandalwood, amber, musk, oakmoss*

White Shoulders is an enduring floral, as charming today as when it was introduced. The predominant note is tuberose; sweet, delicate and feminine, with a soft powdery finish. It is a timeless, tenacious fragrance, attractively priced; now distributed by Parfums International.

Legend has it that White Shoulders was inspired by a baron's love for a woman with exquisite porcelain shoulders, the woman whose cameo still embellishes each pink package.

White Shoulders whispers of a bygone era, of daring low-cut ball gowns, billowing satin and rustling taffeta. An intoxicating scent, it enchants each new generation.

Introduced   1935
Price   Mid-range

WINGS

Scent Type
  Floral - Oriental
Composition
  Top Notes: Ginger lily, green osmanthus, passion flower, gardenia, marigold, blue rose
  Heart Notes: Cattleya orchid, shaffali jasmine, heliotrope
  Base Notes: Woods, amber, musk

This free-spirited composition from the Giorgio-Avon stable was inspired by the "Winged Victory" sculpture at the Louvre museum in Paris. Wings consists of 621 ingredients, blended to evoke spontaneity, positiveness and exhilaration. The result is a delicate balance of sprightly top notes and warm drydown notes. A crisp, invigorating fragrance with a soothing melody, ideal for career days and casual evenings, for the woman who knows no boundaries.

The graceful glass bottle is topped with a blue stopper to represent clear blue sky. Look for the tall statue of a woman with arms outstretched at the Wings beauty counter—she is affectionately nicknamed Ashley and is meant to encourage women to let their spirits soar.

Introduced   1992
Price   Mid-range

...WITH LOVE

Scent Type
  Floral - Oriental
Composition
  Top Notes: Tangerine, black currant bud
  Heart Notes: Jasmine, rose, tuberose, orange blossom, tagetes
  Base Notes: Patchouli, sandalwood, vetiver, musk, amber, labdanum

A floral Oriental with a vibrant fruity top note, ...with Love is the jewel of Fred Hayman's fragrance empire, inspired by the 1990s rebirth of love and renewed commitment.

Rich florals surround smooth fruity top notes of sweet tangerine and black currant bud. The Oriental base notes of mellow woods and amber combine to create a subtle lingering aura. The sophisticated fragrance is suitable for fine affairs, say, lunch at the Bistro Garden in Beverly Hills, not far from Hayman's 273 Rodeo Drive boutique.

Composed by Hayman and a leading French perfumer, the fragrance was also reviewed by Hayman's VIP Fragrance Panel, which includes actress Jean (Mrs. Casey) Kasem, Altovise (Mrs. Sammy) Davis, Victoria (former Mrs. Ed) McMahon, former Beverly Hills mayor Annabelle Heiferman, Beverly Sassoon, singer Jermaine Jackson and his wife Margaret, talk show host and former Miss America Tawny Little, and a number of other women active in fundraising and the cultural and performing arts.

The romantic perfume is ensconced in a rectangular crystal flacon, crowned with a frosted stopper. It is dressed in Hayman's signature colors of red, yellow and gold.

...with Love is a tribute to the 1990s return of romance. Of course, romance never really goes out of style.

Introduced   1991
Price   Top range

WOMENSWEAR
BY
ALEXANDER JULIAN

Scent Type
  Floral
Composition
  Top Notes: *Mandarin, black currant bud, ylang-ylang*
  Heart Notes: *Jasmine, narcissus*
  Base Notes: *Sandalwood, white musk, vanilla*

From renowned menswear designer Alexander Julian comes Womenswear, a fragrance he created for the women who purchase his menswear for their men. Womenswear is a refined floral, resonating with accords of mandarin, black currant bud, jasmine and white musk. Feminine, romantic, elegant. The soft scent is designed to surround a woman with an "aura of scent," never overpowering.

Womenswear is housed in collectible bottles inspired by antique Tuscany jars. Designed by Robert Dugrenier and Meagan (Mrs. Alexander) Julian, the opaque jars are available in iridescent hues of rose, teal or orchid...colors that reflect the essence of Julian himself. Each bottle is an individual work of art, handcrafted for an antiqued sea-glass appearance, resulting in unique color and texture variations. Simply gorgeous.

And finally, Julian gave great attention to making sure the fragrance and packaging are ecologically acceptable. Womenswear was developed without animal testing, paints are lead free, and outer packaging is made from recycled paper.

Introduced   1992
Price   Mid-range

WRAPPINGS

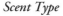

Scent Type
> *Chypre - Green*

Composition
> **Top Notes:** *Sage, artemisia, basil, lavender, mace, aldehydes*
> **Heart Notes:** *Jasmine, cyclamen, hyacinth, lily of the valley, orris, carnation*
> **Base Notes:** *Vetiver, oakmoss, cypress, cedarwood, patchouli, leather, marine*

Wrappings is a fresh green chypre blend from Clinique. The beribboned fragrance has herbal top notes balanced by a heart of white florals and a woody base, with a hint of sea breeze. Wrappings is ideal anytime you want a light, natural scent. Spritz it on for an afternoon of springtime gardening.

Introduced	*1990*
Price	*Mid-range*

Y

Scent Type
> *Chypre - Fruity*

Composition
> **Top Notes:** *Greens, aldehydes, peach, gardenia, mirabelle, honeysuckle*
> **Heart Notes:** *Bulgarian rose, jasmine, tuberose, ylang-ylang, orris, hyacinth*
> **Base Notes:** *Oakmoss, amber, patchouli, sandalwood, vetiver, civet, benzoin, styrax*

Y was the first fragrance introduced by couturier Yves Saint Laurent. Completely different from his later flamboyant creations, Opium and Paris, Y is a light fragrance, delicate, feminine and subtle. A fruity chypre with greens and woods, it is perfect for warm days and active wear.

Introduced	*1964*
Price	*High range*

YOUTH DEW

Scent Type
> *Oriental - Ambery Spicy*

Composition
> **Top Notes:** *Orange, bergamot, peach, spices*
> **Heart Notes:** *Clove, cinnamon, cassie, rose, ylang-ylang, orchid, jasmine*
> **Base Notes:** *Frankincense, amber, vanilla, oakmoss, clove, musk, patchouli, vetiver, spices*

Famous Patrons
  Madonna
  Gloria Swanson
  Joan Crawford
  Dolores Del Rio
  Duchess of Windsor

Youth Dew was the first fragrance produced by Estée Lauder and became the first sensational American fragrance hit when it was introduced as a bath oil for everyday use. During World War II, perfume had been difficult to obtain, and American women were not accustomed to using fragrance every day. They did use bath oils, though, and Lauder seized upon this, marketing her new scent as a bath oil and perfume. She often hinted that Youth Dew was based on a formula her uncle had created for a Russian princess. Women (and men) were swept away by the mystery and the spicy, heady fragrance, and daily fragrance use grew.

The opulent scent has endured as one of Estée Lauder's most popular fragrances. Now available in a wide line of products, Youth Dew is a strong, long-lasting scent, perfect for cool weather and dramatic evenings...or anytime you want to be noticed.

Introduced	*1953*
Price	*Mid-range*

YSATIS

Scent Type
  Chypre - Floral Animalic
Composition
  Top Notes: *Mandarin, bergamot, ylang-ylang, galbanum, orange blossom, coconut, rosewood, greens, aldehydes*
  Heart Notes: *Rose, jasmine, polianthes, iris, tuberose, ylang-ylang, carnation, narcissus*
  Base Notes: *Bay rum, vetiver, patchouli, oakmoss, sandalwood, clove, vanilla, amber, musk, honey, civet, castoreum*

Ysatis is another best-selling fragrance from the House of Givenchy. Pronounce the name "ee-sah-tees." The chypre floral composition unfolds with fruity top notes, followed by an exotic floral accord and warm base notes. Givenchy once described the fragrance as having a "seductive charm." Easy to wear, sophisticated, not overpowering. Ysatis is versatile enough to follow a woman through a busy day from morning meetings to evening interludes. Look for it in a columnar Art Deco-inspired flacon designed by Pierre Dinand.

Introduced	*1985*
Price	*High range*

ZAROLIA

Scent Type
Floral

Composition
Top Notes: *Bulgarian rose, jasmine, lily of the valley*
Heart Notes: *Sandalwood, cedarwood, vetiver*
Base Notes: *Oakmoss*

Famous Patrons
Barbara Bush

Zarolia is a lavish floral composition poised against fragrant woods and mosses.

Conceived as a collectible fragrance by creator Maitland-Phillipe, Zarolia is presented in a variety of containers. One is an exquisite round bottle of frosted glass, topped with a gold-colored cap. The *pièce de résistance* is a handblown art glass flacon, created by designer John Gilvey in the Tiffany manner, signed and dated amidst swirls of amber, violet, gold and turquoise. These one-of-a-kind bottles are specially priced. In fact, Barclay president Ed Elliott says that one is valued at $50,000. But whatever the value of bottle, the priceless fragrance remains the same in each.

Introduced   *1981*
Price   *Top range*

ZIBELINE

Scent Type
Floral - Aldehyde

Composition
Top Notes: *Rose, ylang-ylang, aldehydes*
Heart Notes: *Orange blossom, moss, labdanum*
Base Notes: *Vanilla, benzoin, ambergris*

The word "zibeline" refers to a silky sable pelt, as smooth and precious as the fragrance. Zibeline is another enduring Weil couture fragrance from the Roaring Twenties. Perhaps your grandmother wore Zibeline. But of course, everything old is new again...and Zibeline wouldn't have lasted this long unless it was appreciated.

Fresh florals and aldehydes begin the scent, which evolves into rich floral heart with a dash of spice. Woody balsamics leave an inviting residue, warming the skin like a furry sable coat.

Zibeline can be found swathed in golden shades, standing next to other Weil classics such as Weil de Weil, Antilope and Secret of Venus, all fit for discovery by a new generation.

Introduced   *1928*
Price   *Mid-range*

HONORABLE MENTIONS

The new, the unusual, the hard to find—fragrances "on the cusp" that we wanted to include somewhere. Perhaps they are in limited distribution, or may have just changed distributors. Perhaps they are borderline "prestige perfumes," not quite making our image, pricing or distribution guidelines. Or maybe the company didn't reply to our inquiries, or we simply couldn't find complete information.

Whatever the story, we didn't want you to go mad thinking, "I once fell in love with a fragrance, it must be here somewhere!" We've included all we could, more than sixty fragrances in these Honorable Mentions.

If you have the inside track on any of these or others, drop us a line—we'd love to hear from you so that we make our next book even better.

Fragrance	House/Distributor	Scent Type
Action	Trussardi	Floral - Green
Adolfo	Trend Media	Floral
Aria Missoni	Orlane	Floral - Ambery
Bambou	Weil	Floral - Fruity
Baruffa	Atkinsons	Floral - Fruity
Bibi	Cofci	Chypre - Floral
Bizarre	Atkinsons	Floral - Green
Blue Paradise	MCM	Floral - Fruity
Café	French Fragrances	Semi-Oriental
Capucci	Capucci	Chypre - Floral
Clandestine	Larouche	Floral - Ambery
Climat	Lancôme	Floral - Oriental
Daniel de Fasson	Parlux	Floral - Oriental
Dans la Nuit	Worth	Floral - Oriental
Deneuve	Phénix	Floral - Green
Dynamisante	Clarins	Chypre
Eau de Caron	Caron	Oriental - Ambery
Eau d'Orlane	Orlane	Floral - Fruity
Echo	Mario Valentino	Floral
Euforia	Atkinsons	Floral - Fresh
Experiences	P. Presley/Muelhens	TBA*
Fantasme	Ted Lapidus	Floral - Fruity
Filly	Capucci	Floral
Fleurs d'Orlane	Orlane	Floral - Fresh
Glorious	Vanderbilt/Cosmair	Floral

Issey Miyake	Issey Miyake	Floral - Fruity
J'ai Osé	Laroche	Oriental - Ambery
Jaïs	Atkinsons	Floral - Fruity
Jungle Gardenia	Tuvaché	Floral
Kenzo Parfum d'Ete	Kenzo	Floral - Oriental
Krazy Krizia	Krizia	Oriental
Lancaster	Lancaster	Oriental - Ambery
Lyra	Parfums Alain Delon	Floral - Ambery
Maja	Myrurgia	Fougère
Mariel by M. Hemingway	H20 Stores	Floral - Fruity
Maxim's de Paris	Maxim's	Floral - Aldehyde
Métal	Compar	Floral - Aldehyde
Misha	Barrie	Chypre - Floral Animalic
Missoni	Orlane	Chypre - Floral
Molto Missoni	Orlane	Oriental - Ambery
1900	MCM	Floral - Ambery
Norma Kamali	Kamali	Floral - Ambery
Ô Intense	Lancôme	Floral - Oriental
Ô de Lancôme	Lancôme	Chypre - Fresh
Obelisk	MCM	Oriental - Ambery
Ombre Bleue	Brosseau/J. Phillipe	Floral
Ombre de la Nuit	Ungaro	Oriental - Spicy
Only	Julio Iglesias	Floral - Ambery
Outrageous Watne	Watne	Floral
Prada	Orlane	Chypre - Floral
Présence	Parfums Parquet	Floral
Privilège	Privilège	Floral
Rapture	Victoria's Secret	Floral - Oriental
Regine's	Jean Phillipe	Fruity Floral
Samba Nova	Perfumer's Workshop	Oriental
Shocking	Schiaparelli	Oriental - Ambery Spicy
Shu Uemura	Uemura	Floral - Ambery
Silences	Jacomo	Floral - Green
Soir de Paris	Bourjois	Floral
Todd Oldham	Parlux	TBA*
Ugo Vanelli	TBA*	Floral - Fruity
U II	Ultima	Chypre - Green
Victoria	Victoria's Secret	Floral
Vivage Jour	Louis Férand	Floral - Fresh
Yendi	Capucci	Floral

TBA = To Be Announced. Information not available at time of print.

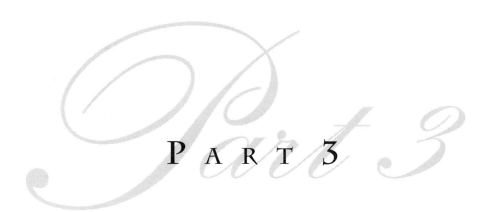

PART 3

PROFILE FRAGRANCES BY SCENT TYPE

FLORAL

Adoration
Anne Klein
Antonia's Flowers
Azzaro 9
Beautiful
Bellodgia
Bill Blass
Bulgari Eau Parfumée
Capricci
Carolina Herrera
Catalyst
Celia's Ultimate Gardenia
Channel No. 22
Chloé
Coeur-Joie
Courrèges in Blue
Delicious
Demi-Jour
Diamonds and Emeralds
Dilys
Donna Karan New York
EarthSource - Windfresh Flowers
Eau du Ciel
Ecco
Ellen Tracy
Estée
Evelyn
Fidji
Fleurs de Rocaille
Fracas
Fred Hayman's Touch
Gabriela Sabatini
Gardenia
Gardénia Passion
Gianfranco Ferre
Giorgio Beverly Hills
Golconda
Heure Exquise

Ice Water by Pino Silvestre
Isis
Jardins de Bagatelle
Joy
K de Krizia
Kenzo
L'Air du Temps
L'Insolent
Lalique
Les Fleurs de Claude Monet
Lumière
Mad Moments
Madeleine de Madeleine
Maud Frizon Parfum
Michelle
Nina
Niro 15
Niro 119
Noir for Women by Pascal Morabito
Norell
One Perfect Rose
1000 de Jean Patou
One Unlimited - Malaga
One Unlimited - Mandalay
One Unlimited - Provence
Paris
Passion
Pavlova
Quadrille
Quelques Fleurs L'Original
Red Door
Rose Absolue
Scaasi
Society by Burberrys
Spoiled
Tatiana
360 Perry Ellis
Tubéreuse
273 for Women

Un Jour
Vicky Tiel
Vivid
Volcan D'Amour
Vôtre
White Diamonds
White Shoulders
Womenswear by Alexander Julian
Zarolia

FLORAL - GREEN

Andiamo
Cabotine
Chanel No. 19
Eau de Camille
Fleurs d'Elle
Ivoire
Jessica McClintock
Léonard de Léonard
Safari
Sung, Alfred Sung
Vent Vert
Weil de Weil

FLORAL - FRUITY

Adieu Sagesse - Ma Collection
Amarige
Amazone
Basic Black
Byblos
Calyx
Champagne
Design
Diamonds and Sapphires
EarthSource - Sunwarmed Peach
Eau d'Hermès
Eau de Charlotte
Eau de Givenchy
Elysium

Escape
Ferre by Ferre
Folavril
Genny Shine
Giò
Il Bacio
Jean-Paul Gaultier
La Prairie
Laura Ashley No. 1
Lauren
Listen
Liz Claiborne
Magnetic
Molinard de Molinard
Nicole Miller (aura-floral)
One Unlimited - Capri
Quartz
Romeo Gigli
Senso
Smalto Donna
Sunflowers
Sweet Courrèges
Tribù
Versus for Women

FLORAL - FRESH

Amour Amour - Ma Collection
Anaïs Anaïs
Câline - Ma Collection
Destiny
Diorissimo
EarthSource - Rainswept Jasmine
Eau de Gucci
Eternity
Laguna
Moods
Tendre Poison

FLORAL - ALDEHYDE

Antilope
Arpège
Bois des Îles
Calandre
Calèche
Channel No. 5

Farouche
First
Fleur de Fleurs
Gucci No. 1
Infini
Je Reviens
L'Intredit
Le Dix
Liu
Lutéce
Madame Rochas
My Sin
Nahema
Nocturnes
Nude
Ombre Rose
Red
Rive Gauche
Salvador Dali
Scherrer 2
Tamango
White Linen
Zibeline

FLORAL - AMBERY

Après L'Ondée
Balahé
Blue Grass
C'est la vie!
Caesars Woman
DNA
L'Heure Bleue
Mademoiselle Ricci
Moment Suprême - Ma Collection
Oscar de la Renta
Panthère
Poison
Spellbound
Tiffany

FLORAL - OCEANIC

Dune

FLORAL ORIENTAL

Alfred Sung E.N.C.O.R.E.
Asja
Bijan
Charles of the Ritz
Chloé Narcisse
Coco
Di Borghese
Diamonds and Rubies
Dolce & Gabbana
Escada by Margaretha Ley
Fiamma
Galanos
Galore
Jil Sander No. 4
Joop! pour Femme
Mackie, Bob Mackie
Maroussia
Moschino
Narcisse Noir
One Unlimited - Indochine
Raffinée
Realities
Rose Cardin
Samsara
Secret of Venus
Tuscany per Donna
Vacances - Ma Collection
Van Cleef & Arpels
Vanderbilt
Vendetta
Venezia
Volupté
Wings
...with Love

FLORAL SEMI-ORIENTAL

Boucheron
Byzance
Chamade
Désirade
Elizabeth Taylor's Passion
Trésor

SEMI-ORIENTAL
Alexandra
Colors de Benetton
Parfum d'Hermès
Sonia Rykiel

ORIENTAL
Angel
Chaldée - Ma Collection
Coquette
Hot
Nuit de Noël
Odalisque
Oh la la!
Realm
Royal Secret
Shalimar

ORIENTAL - AMBERY
Anne Klein II
Chantilly
Ciara
Dionne
Divine Folie - Ma Collection
Guess?
Habanita
Must de Cartier
Normandie - Ma Collection
Obsession
Roma
Ungaro

ORIENTAL - FRUITY
Casmir

ORIENTAL - SPICY
Cinnabar
Dioressence
KL
L'Heure Attendue - Ma Collection
Ma Liberté
Opium
Parfum Sacré
Prélude
Teatro alla Scala
Tianne

ORIENTAL - AMBERY SPICY
Bal à Versailles
Magie Noire
Vol de Nuit
Youth Dew

CHYPRE
Enigma
Feminité du Bois

CHYPRE - FRUITY
Azzaro
Cocktail - Ma Collection
Colony - Ma Collection
Femme
Gem
Mitsouko
Que sais-je? - Ma Collection
Y

CHYPRE - FRUITY FLORAL
Cassini by Oleg Cassini

CHYPRE - FLORAL ANIMALIC
Azurée
Bandit
Cabochard
Cuir de Russie
Empreinte
Givenchy III
Jolie Madame
Miss Balmain
Miss Dior
Moments by Priscilla Presley
Mystère
Parure
Rumba
Ysatis

CHYPRE - FLORAL
Animale
Aromatics Elixir
Chant d'Arômes
Coriandre
Diva
Fendi

Gucci No. 3
Halston
Histoire D'Amour
Knowing
L'Arte de Gucci
Ma Griffe
Montana Parfum de Peau
Niki de Saint Phalle
Paloma Picasso
V'E Versace

CHYPRE - FRESH
Création
Cristalle
Diorella
Eau d'Hadrien
Eau de Rochas
4711 Eau de Cologne

CHYPRE - GREEN
Aliage
Private Collection
Wrappings

CITRUS
Eau de Cologne du Coq
Eau de Cologne Hermès
Eau de Cologne Impériale
Eau de Guerlain
Eau de Patou
Eau Fraîche by Léonard

GREEN
Alfred Sung Spa
One Unlimited - Emerald Isle
Pheromone
Reverie

FOUGÈRE
Jicky

COMMONLY USED INGREDIENTS IN PERFUMERY
For ingredients not listed, consult a dictionary or encyclopedia.

Aldehydes - Organic chemicals derived from natural or synthetic materials. Aldehydes add a vivid, quick quality to top notes. Variations can be powdery, fruity, green, citrusy, floral or woody.

Amber - A fossil resin from the fir tree. Prized for its tenacity, it also adds warm, leathery, powdery elements to a composition. The color amber refers to the color of the resin.

Ambergris - Secretion from the male sperm whale, often found floating in the ocean. The Chinese once used it as an aphrodisiac. Ambergris imparts a woody, balsamic odor. Substitutes are used more often today, because the natural substance is difficult to obtain.

Ambrette Seed - These plant seeds yield a musky floral, brandy-type aroma.

Anjelica - Oil from the root of the angelica tree, which is cultivated in France, Belgium and Germany. It is musky and peppery, with a spicy green quality.

Balsam - Tree resins that exhibit a warm, sweet element. They are generally used as a base fixative.

Basil - A spicy herb with a green impression.

Bay Leaf - A tree leaf valued for its spicy, warm, almost bitter scent.

Bayberry - A shrub with berries, from which a waxy substance is taken. Bayberry adds a spicy, woody flair to fragrance.

Benzoin - Balsamic resin from the tropical styrax tree, used as a fixative, imparting a sweet, cocoa-like quality. Benzoin is found in Thailand, Vietnam and Laos.

Bergamot - Oil produced from the peel of the bergamot fruit. The inedible fruit is of the citrus family and is about the size of an orange. The largest bergamot production comes from Calabria, Italy. The fresh, citrus essence is ideal in top notes and eau de cologne.

Black Currant Bud - (*see Cassis*)

Boronia - Essence taken from the flower of the boronia bush, which is mainly found in Australia. Often used in chypre blends, it leaves a spicy-rosy impression.

Broom - This produces a sweet, grassy odor. It is derived from the blossoms of the Mediterranean-area Spanish broom shrub.

Buchu - Substance from the leaves of the buchu herb. It yields a strong minty, camphor odor.

Bulgarian Rose - A highly valued flower in perfumery, grown in Bulgaria's Valley of the Roses at the base of the Balkan mountain range, where a Turkish merchant began cultivation centuries ago.

Cardamom - Oil distilled from the cardamom plant, a member of the ginger family. It leaves a spicy floral impression. It is second only to saffron as the world's most expensive spice. In India, cardamom grains are chewed to freshen the breath.

Carnation - This flower gives off a spicy, sensual aroma.

Cassia Oil - Obtained from the leaves of an evergreen tree, valued for its spicy cinnamon-like quality. The oil is also used in cola drinks.

Cassie - Derived from the Acacia farnesiana bush, the cassie absolute produces a spicy floral flavor.

Cassis - Oil taken from the bud of the black currant fruit, which is also used in liqueur.

Castoreum - A secretion from the beaver that exudes a leathery quality and is used as a fixative.

Cedarwood - Oil obtained from the juniper cedar tree, which is native to Texas. An excellent fixative, it has a distinct wood tone.

Chamomile - A sweet, herbal odor with fruity notes, often used to balance floral compositions.

Cinnamon - Oil obtained from the bark and leaves of the cinnamomum tree, which is native to Southeast Asia and the East Indies. It imparts a familiar warm, sweet, spicy odor.

Civet - A glandular secretion from the civet cat, used as a fixative. Repugnant by itself, civet blends well and adds a warm, leathery, erotic tone to a composition.

Clary Sage - An herb valued for its sweet, subtle quality.

Clove - Obtained from the clove tree, clove buds are prized for their spicy sweetness. The tree is cultivated in Sri Lanka, Madagascar and Indonesia.

Coriander - Oil from the coriander herb of the parsley family, valued for its spicy aromatic impression.

Costus - Essence from the root of the costus plant of the daisy family, lends warmth to Oriental blends. It has green, violet-like accents.

Coumarin - Obtained from the tonka bean and often created synthetically, produces a sweet, herbal, spicy, hay-like odor, similar to vanilla.

Cyclamen - Essence taken from the heart-shaped flowers of the primrose family.

Eucalyptus - Oil from the leaves of the eucalyptus tree, leaves a strong herbal, camphor impression. Discovered in Tasmania, it is widely cultivated in Spain, Portugal and Australia and is well priced.

Frangipani - Oil from the sweet, jasmine-like flowers of the frangipani tree.

Frankincense (*see Olibanum*)

Galbanum - A gum resin valued for its leafy green, soft balsamic odor. Galbanum is used in many fragrances to provide a pleasing freshness, or green lift.

Gardenia - A heady white flower with a strong sweet scent.

Geranium - Oil made from the leaves and stems of the plant. Depending on the variety, it gives off a rosy, minty or fruity essence often used in rosy or spicy compositions.

Ginger - A woody, warm, spicy odor derived from the ginger plant.

Gums - Resins or balsams secreted from plants. Exhibiting a sweet tenacious odor, they are often used as fixatives.

Heliotropin - An aldehyde with a floral almond tone, found in pepper oil.

Honeysuckle - A highly fragrant vine flower but difficult to capture correctly. The essence of honeysuckle is usually re-created by blending a variety of florals.

Hyacinth - A sweet floral that imparts a green impression.

Incense - Made from gums and resins, produces a spicy aroma when burned.

Jasmine - Called the king of flowers, a sweet tiny white flower with a vibrant, smooth aroma. Jasmine is one of the most prized essences in the perfumer's palette. It is grown in France, Morocco, India, Egypt and Spain and must be harvested before sunrise to retain the full amount of its delicate fragrance.

Jonquil - Highly fragrant essence derived from a flower of the narcissus family, rare because it is difficult to distill.

Labdanum - A dark resin obtained from the rockrose herb, valued for its leathery odor.

Lavender - From the flowering tops of lavender plants in France, Spain, Morocco and old Yugoslavia, a sweet, light essence with woody floral accents. The oil is used in lavender waters, chypres, fougères and florals. Lavender water is said to have been a favorite of Madame de Pompadour, mistress of Louis XV.

Leather - A smoky, sweet, animal odor crafted from the perfumer's palette. It is warm and persistent.

Lemon - Oil from the lemon rind. It is a zesty, sharp, refreshing essence, and is added to brighten many compositions, particularly eau de cologne.

Lilac - Since the essence released by the lilac plant and flower does not accurately portray its aroma, the perfumer re-creates the essence by using jasmine, ylang-ylang, neroli and vanilla.

Lily of the Valley - Also known as muguet, lily of the valley is invented by the perfumer, using jasmine, orange blossom, rose, ylang-ylang and chemical additives. The sweet essence is difficult to obtain from the natural flower.

Magnolia - A sweet, highly fragrant flower, also stubborn in releasing its essence. The perfumer re-creates the essence by blending rose, jasmine, neroli and ylang-ylang with aroma chemicals.

Mandarin - Oil from the peel of the mandarin orange fruit, a brisk, sweet essence often used in eau de cologne.

May Rose - Also called rose de mai. The May rose from Morocco produces a rich, long-lasting oil prized for its full-bodied, diffusive qualities.

Mimosa - A green floral essence obtained from mimosa tree flowers and stems. It imparts a smooth, sweet aroma.

Moss - Earthy essences are derived from a variety of mosses: oakmoss, treemoss, lichen, seaweed and algae.

Muguet (*see Lily of the Valley*)

Musk - A glandular secretion from the male musk deer of Tibet, China and Nepal, used as a fixative in fine perfumes. It is valued for its woody, animal, erotic impressions, though nowadays it is often created chemically by the perfumer. Soft, sensuous, pervasive.

Narcissus - A highly fragrant yellow and white flower that produces an intense spicy, earthy and sweet straw-like odor. Small amounts are often used to round off floral compositions. Native to Persia, the narcissus flower was carried to China over the silk route in the eighth century.

Neroli - Made from the orange blossoms of the bitter orange tree grown in France, Egypt, Algeria and Morocco. It is light, sweet and spicy and is used in top notes and eau de cologne. It was named for the Duchess of Nerola and was often used to scent gloves.

Nutmeg - Spicy oil derived from the seeds of the South Asian nutmeg tree.

Oakmoss - A lichen grown on oak trees. Its odor is earthy, woody and slightly leathery. It is used as a fixative in many blends, especially chypre.

Olibanum - Also called frankincense. Olibanum is a gum resin from a tree found in Africa and Saudia Arabia. An outstanding fixative, its odor is spicy and balsamic, similar to that of incense.

Opopanax - Derived from a gum resin and similar to myrrh. A woody, sweet fixative.

Orange Blossom - From the white blossoms of the bitter orange tree. It adds a warm, spicy flavor that is often used in floral compositions.

Orange Oil - Produced from the peel of the orange, and often used in eau de cologne and floral fragrances. Refreshing, sweet, fruity and crisp.

Orris - One of the most expensive ingredients used in perfumery. It is obtained from the iris plant, which is commonly cultivated in Italy. Its odor is violet-like and can be warm, sweet, woody, fruity or floral, depending on the quality.

Osmanthus - Produced from the flowers of the osmanthus tree, which is found in Japan, China and Southeast Asia. It has a floral odor, with a hint of plum and raisin.

Patchouli - Oil obtained from the leaves of the patchouli plant, a superb fixative. Discovered in India, it is also cultivated in Malaysia and Indonesia. Its odor is earthy, dry, woody and spicy. Patchouli is often used in Oriental and chypre blends.

Petitgrain - Essence derived from the leaves and stems of the bitter orange tree. It has a subtle woody tone similar to neroli. Sweet and floral, petitgrain adds freshness to a fragrance, especially eau de cologne.

Resin - Gum secretions from trees and plants, often used as fixatives.

Rose - Rose oil is also referred to as "otto" or "attar" of rose; these terms refer to perfume oil produced through distillation. There is a wide variety of roses, and the rich oil they produce has the familiar rose aroma, though undertones vary from honey to fruity, spicy to musk, and violet to green. Called the queen of flowers, it is one of the most precious ingredients in perfumery. Roses bloom just thirty days of the year and must be picked quickly, for they lose half their essence by noon. Centifolia and

Damascena are popularly cultivated roses. The floral essence is used in rose water, floral, chypre and Oriental compositions. Rose water was said to have been a favorite of Marie Antoinette.

Rose de Mai (*see May Rose*)

Rosemary - Flowers and leaves of the evergreen rosemary herb of the mint family, distilled for use in perfumery. The oil produces an herbal note that is woody and slightly lavender-like.

Rosewood Oil - Oil obtained from the wood of the rosewood tree, the aniba rosaeodora of the laurel family. It gives off a rosy odor, sweet and subtly spicy. Rosewood is often added to eau de cologne.

Sage - A fresh, spicy odor from the sage herb.

Sandalwood - Oil from the sandalwood tree, the evergreen santalum album grown in India, Australia and Southeast Asia, though the Indian province of Mysore supplies 85% of all sandalwood. The wood is valued for its aroma and its imperviousness to termites. The trees must mature at least thirty years for the oil to fully develop. An expensive ingredient, sandalwood oil is prized for its fixative quality. Its odor is powdery, balsamic, woody and rich. Sandalwood gives a smooth finish to Oriental, chypre and floral perfumes.

Styrax - A sweet balsam found on the styrax tree, an excellent fixative.

Sweet Pea - A flower oil produced from the fragrant flowering vine, valued for its light, delicate nature.

Tagetes - Essence produced from the tagetes flower, which is grown in Spain, Italy and South Africa. The strong essence has an herbal, aromatic personality with fruity undertones.

Thyme - Derived from the flowering herb. Thyme smells sweet and herbaceous—ideal for eau de cologne.

Tonka Bean - Fragrant seeds from native South American trees of the Dipteryx family.

Tuberose - One of the most expensive oils, from a flower known for its rich, sensual aroma. Its cost is due in part to a painstaking processing called enfleurage, an oil extraction method whereby the flowers are pressed into

fat, then the oil is separated with alcohol. Tuberose is a perennial plant native to Mexico. The sweet, honey-like aroma adds fullness to many floral fragrances and blends well with gardenia, jonquil and hyacinth.

Vanilla - Made from the fruit and seeds of a climbing orchid vine. It has pods, or capsules encasing the beans. Vanilla is an impressive sweet fixative, used in many Oriental, amber and floral perfumes.

Vanillin - Can be produced naturally from the vanilla pod, and from certain balsams and benzoins. It can also be made synthetically. Its sweet, strong odor is similar to vanilla, but lacks the depth of vanilla. Vanillin blends well with vanilla to produce a round, full-bodied vanilla aroma.

Vetiver - A grass grown in Haiti, Réunion Island, Brazil, China and Southeast Asia. It has a woody, earthy quality, enhanced by a moist balsamic accent. A superb fixative, vetiver is an important component in chypre blends.

Violet - The violet flower yields such a minute amount of oil that it is cost prohibitive to extract. Instead, the violet aroma is created chemically for use in perfumery.

Violet Leaf - Oil from the leaves of the violet plant, valued for its cucumbery green and peppery herbal aroma, with touches of violet and iris. Parma, Italy, is known for its violet production.

Ylang-Ylang - From Tagalog for "flower of flowers." This oil comes from the flower of ylang-ylang trees grown in Madagascar, Indonesia, Comoros and the Philippines. The rich oil has a jasmine-like aroma and sweet balsamic accents. Used in many floral and Oriental compositions, ylang-ylang smooths and rounds bitter notes, adding warmth and grace.

BIBLIOGRAPHY AND SOURCES

"The Effect of Fragrance on the Mood of a Woman at Midlife," "Mood Benefits of Fragrance." *Aroma-Chology Review*, Vol. II, No. 1.

Beauty Fashion. January 1991 through January 1994.

Bork, Karl-Heinz; Elke Doerrier; Arturetto Landi; Egon Oelkers; Peter Woerner; Lothar Kuemper. *Fragrance Guide: Feminine Notes, Masculine Notes.* Hamburg, Germany: Glöss Verlag, 1991.

Science & Technology. "No One's Sniffing at Aroma Research Now." *Business Week,* December 23, 1991, 82.

Chanel, Inc. *Chanel Fragrances.* New York: Chanel, Inc., 1991.

"How to Buy a Fragrance." *Consumer Reports,* December 1993, 765-773.

"All Passion Scent." *Country Living.*

"The Raison d'être of the Fragrance Foundation: Past, Present and Future." *Dragoco Report,* January 1991, 3-9.

Etherington-Smith, Meredith. *Patou.* New York: St. Martin's, 1983.

Fischer-Rizzi, Susanne. *Complete Aromatherapy Handbook: Essential Oils for Radiant Health.* New York: Sterling Publishing, 1990.

The Fragrance Foundation. *The Facts and Fun of Fragrance.* New York: Fragrance Foundation, 1992.

The Fragrance Foundation. *Fragrance and Olfactory Directory.* New York: Fragrance Foundation, 1981.

The Fragrance Foundation. *The History, the Mystery, the Enjoyment of Fragrance.* New York: Fragrance Foundation.

Gaborit, Jean-Yves. *Perfumes: The Essences and Their Bottles.* New York: Rizzoli, 1985.

Israel, Lee. *Estée Lauder: Beyond the Magic.* New York: MacMillan Publishing Co., 1985.

Kaufman, William. *Perfume.* New York: E.P. Dutton & Co., 1974.

"History of an Ancient Art," "Lalique Parfums," "Recipe for a Fragrance." *Lalique Magazine,* Winter 1993, 4-11.

Lauder, Estée. *Estée: A Success Story.* New York: Random House, 1985.

"Scientists Say Aromas Have Major Effect on Emotions." *Los Angeles Times,* May 31, 1991, B3.

Monroe, Valerie. "How to Smell Really Wonderful." *McCall's,* September 1993, 140, 182.

"Scent System." *Mirabella,* October 1991, 142-143.

Morris, Edwin T. *Fragrance: The Story of Perfume from Cleopatra to Chanel.* New York: Charles Scribner's Sons, 1984.

Müller, Julia. *The H&R Book of Perfume.* Hamburg, Germany: Glöss Verlag, 1992.

"The Intimate Sense." *National Geographic,* September 1986, 324-360.

"Discovery May Unlock Secret of Smell." *New York Times,* April 5, 1991, A1.

Ohrbach, Barbara Milo. *A Bouquet of Flowers: Sweet Thoughts, Recipes, and Gifts from the Garden with "The Language of Flowers."* New York: Clarkson N. Potter, Inc., 1990.

Olfactory Research Fund Ltd. *Living Well With Your Sense of Smell.* New York: Olfactory Research Fund Ltd., 1992.

"Dollars and Scents." *Philadelphia Inquirer,* September 29, 1991, section J.

Pickles, Sheila. *The Language of Flowers.* New York: Harmony Books, 1989.

"The Coming Age of Aroma-Chology." *Soap/Cosmetics/Chemical Specialties,* April 1991, 30-32.

Von Furstenberg, Diane. *Diane von Fürstenberg's Book of Beauty.* New York: Simon & Schuster, 1976.

Lab Notes. "Sniffing Heliotrope Helps MRI Patients Sit Still." *Wall Street Journal,* August 8, 1991.

"What the Nose Knows." *Washington Post,* July 26, 1992.

Green, Annette; Fragrance Foundation. Interviewed by author. October 1993.

Hayman, Gale; Gale Hayman Beverly Hills. Interviewed by author. October 1993.

Mosbacher, Georgette, and Paulsin, Lyn; Exclusives. Interviewed by author. October 1993.

Nance, Bunni; Neiman Marcus. Interviewed by author. August 1993.

Completed questionnaires, interviews, information, permissions, media kits and photography were supplied, in part or in total, by the following companies:

H. Alpert & Company, Laura Ashley, Barclay Perfumes, Benetton Cosmetics, Bijan, Boucheron, Bulgari, Cassini Parfums, Caesars World Merchandising, Chanel, Liz Claiborne, Compar, Cosmair, Dionne Inc., Christian Dior, Erox, Escada, EuroCos, Marilyn Evins, Exclusives, Alice Fixx, The Fragrance Foundation, French Fragrances, Givenchy, Annick Goutal, Guerlain, Fred Hayman, Gale Hayman, Hermès, Donna Karan Beauty Company, Lancaster Group, Ralph Lauren Fragrances, L'Oréal, Marina Maher, Marilyn Miglin, Jessica McClintock, Madeleine Mono, Georgette Mosbacher, Neiman Marcus, Niro, Nordstrom's, Olfactory Research Fund, William Owen, Parfums International, Jean Patou, Perfumania, Prescriptives, Revlon, Riviera Concepts, Rochas, Chen Sam, Paul Sebastian, Tiffany, Ungaro, Vepro and Diane Von Furstenberg.

BUYER'S GUIDE

Some fragrances are exclusive to certain stores while others are widely distributed. For information on where to purchase in your area, contact the distributors or contacts listed below. *(All United States telephone numbers.)*

To submit information for future editions of *Fabulous Fragrances*, write to us at Crescent House Publishing: P.O. Box 16724, Beverly Hills, California, 90209. To order more copies of *Fabulous Fragrances*, see the order card at the back of this book.

Fragrance	Distribution/Contact	Phone
Adieu Sagesse (Ma Collection)	Jean Patou	(212) 688-5568
Adoration	Wm. Owen Fragrances	(407) 833-4076
Alexandra	Alexandra de Markoff/Revlon	(212) 527-4000
Alfred Sung E.N.C.O.R.E.	Sung/Riviera Concepts	(213) 658-7864
Alfred Sung Spa	Sung/Riviera Concepts	(213) 658-7864
Aliage	Estée Lauder	(212) 572-4200
Amarige	Parfums Givenchy	(212) 759-7566
Amazone	Hermes Parfums	(212) 759-7585
Amour Amour	Jean Patou	(212) 688-5568
Anaïs Anaïs	Cacharel/Cosmair	(212) 818-1500
Andiamo	Halston Borghese	(212) 572-3100
Angel	Thierry Mugler	(212) 758-0400
Animale	Parlux Fragrances	(305) 946-7700
Anne Klein	Parlux Fragrances	(305) 946-7700
Anne Klein II	Parlux Fragrances	(305) 946-7700
Antilope	Classic Fragrances Ltd.	(212) 929-2266
Antonia's Flowers	Antonia's Flowers	(516) 324-7103
Après L'Ondée	Guerlain	(212) 751-1870
Aromatics Elixir	Clinique Laboratories	(212) 572-3800
Arpège	L'Oreal/Cosmair	(212) 984-4535
Asja	Fendi/Parfums International	(212) 261-1000
Azurée	Estée Lauder	(212) 572-4200
Azzaro 9	MacFarlane & Associates	(914) 639-9170
Azzaro	MacFarlane & Associates	(914) 639-9170
Bal à Versailles	Desprez/Alfin	(212) 333-7700
Balahé	Léonard/Jean Pax	(305) 593-0982
Bandit	Piguet/Alfin	(212) 333-7700
Basic Black	Blass/Revlon	(212) 527-4000
Beautiful	Estée Lauder	(212) 572-4200
Bellodgia	Caron/Jean Patou	(212) 688-5568
Bijan	Bijan Fragrances	(310) 271-1122
Bill Blass	Blass/Revlon	(212) 527-4000
Blue Grass	Elizabeth Arden Co.	(212) 261-1350
Bois des Îles	Chanel	(212) 688-5055
Boucheron	Boucheron	(212) 688-1610
Bulgari Eau Parfumée	Bulgari	(800) BUL-GARI
Byblos	Gary Farn, Ltd.	(203) 878-8900
Byzance	Rochas/Jean Patou	(212) 688-5568
C'est la vie!	Parfums Christian Lacroix	(212) 751-5144
Cabochard	Grès/Gary Farn, Ltd.	(203) 878-8900
Cabotine	Grès/Gary Farn, Ltd.	(203) 878-8900
Caesars Woman	Caesars World Merchandising	(310) 552-2711
Calandre	Compar	(212) 980-9620

Calèche	Hermes Parfums	(212) 759-7585
Câline (Ma Collection)	Jean Patou	(212) 688-5568
Calyx	Prescriptives	(212) 572-4000
Capricci	Nina Ricci Parfums	(212) 230-0500
Carolina Herrera	Compar	(212) 980-9620
Casmir	Chopard/Lancaster Group	(212) 593-7400
Cassini by Oleg Cassini	Cassini Parfums, Ltd.	(212) 755-3490
Catalyst	Halston Borghese	(212) 572-3100
Celia's Ultimate Gardenia	Wm. Owen Fragrances	(407) 833-4076
Chaldée (Ma Collection)	Jean Patou	(212) 688-5568
Chamade	Guerlain	(212) 751-1870
Champagne	Yves Saint Laurent	(212) 621-7300
Chanel No. 5	Chanel	(212) 688-5055
Chanel No. 19	Chanel	(212) 688-5055
Chanel No. 22	Chanel	(212) 688-5055
Chant d'Arômes	Guerlain	(212) 751-1870
Chantilly	Parquet/Houbigant	(201) 941-3400
Charles of the Ritz	Revlon	(212) 527-4000
Chloé Narcisse	Parfums International	(212) 261-1000
Chloé	Parfums International	(212) 261-1000
Ciara	Revlon	(212) 527-4000
Cinnabar	Estée Lauder	(212) 572-4200
Cocktail (Ma Collection)	Jean Patou	(212) 688-5568
Coco	Chanel	(212) 688-5055
Coeur-Joie	Nina Ricci Parfums	(212) 230-0500
Colony (Ma Collection)	Jean Patou	(212) 688-5568
Colors de Benetton	Benetton Cosmetics Corp.	(212) 832-6616
Coquette	Wm. Owen Fragrances	(407) 833-4076
Coriandre	Classic Fragrances Ltd.	(212) 929-2266
Courrèges in Blue	Courrèges/Jean Pax	(305) 593-0982
Création	Lapidus/Fragrance Group	(212) 557-8177
Cristalle	Chanel	(212) 688-5055
Cuir de Russie	Chanel	(212) 688-5055
Delicious	Gale Hayman Beverly Hills	(212) 754-6666
Demi-Jour	Parfums Houbigant Paris	(201) 945-2666
Design	Paul Sebastian	(908) 493-4499
Destiny	Marilyn Miglin	(312) 943-1120
Désirade	French Fragrances	(305) 624-7849
Di Borghese	Halston Borghese	(212) 572-3100
Diamonds and Emeralds	Taylor/Parfums International	(212) 261-1000
Diamonds and Rubies	Taylor/Parfums International	(212) 261-1000
Diamonds and Sapphires	Taylor/Parfums International	(212) 261-1000
Dilys	Ashley/Alfin	(212) 333-7700
Dionne	Dionne	(608) 271-3736
Diorella	Christian Dior Perfumes	(212) 418-0400
Dioressence	Christian Dior Perfumes	(212) 418-0400
Diorissimo	Christian Dior Perfumes	(212) 418-0400
Diva	Ungaro Parfums	(212) 303-5920
Divine Folie (Ma Collection)	Jean Patou	(212) 688-5568
DNA Perfume by Bijan	Bijan Fragrances	(310) 271-1122
Dolce & Gabbana	H. Alpert & Co.	(310) 478-0222
Donna Karan New York	The Donna Karan Company	(212) 789-1500
Dune	Christian Dior Perfumes	(212) 418-0400
EarthSource	H. Alpert & Co.	(310) 478-0222
Eau d'Hadrien	Annick Goutal	(212) 759-0650
Eau d'Hermès	Hermes Parfums	(212) 759-7585

Eau de Camille	Annick Goutal	(212) 759-0650
Eau de Charlotte	Annick Goutal	(212) 759-0650
Eau de Cologne du Coq	Guerlain	(212) 751-1870
Eau de Cologne Hermès	Hermes Parfums	(212) 759-7585
Eau de Cologne Impériale	Guerlain	(212) 751-1870
Eau de Givenchy	Parfums Givenchy	(212) 759-7566
Eau de Gucci	Gucci/Muelhens	(203) 787-4711
Eau de Guerlain	Guerlain	(212) 751-1870
Eau de Patou	Jean Patou	(212) 688-5568
Eau de Rochas	Rochas/Jean Patou	(212) 688-5568
Eau du Ciel	Annick Goutal	(212) 759-0650
Eau Fraîche by Léonard	Léonard/Jean Pax	(305) 593-0982
Ecco	Halston Borghese	(212) 572-3100
Elizabeth Taylor's Passion	Taylor/Parfums International	(212) 261-1000
Ellen Tracy	Revlon	(212) 527-4000
Elysium	Clarins	(212) 355-7175
Empreinte	Courrèges/Jean Pax	(305) 593-0982
Enigma	Alexandra de Markoff/Revlon	(212) 527-4000
Escada by Margaretha Ley	Escada Beaute	(212) 852-5500
Escape	Calvin Klein Cosmetics	(212) 759-8888
Estée	Estée Lauder	(212) 572-4200
Eternity	Calvin Klein Cosmetics	(212) 759-8888
Evelyn	Crabtree and Evelyn	(800) 624-5211
Farouche	Nina Ricci Parfums	(212) 230-0500
Feminité du Bois	Shiseido Cosmetics Ltd.	(212) 752-2644
Femme	Rochas/Jean Patou	(212) 688-5568
Fendi	Fendi/Parfums International	(212) 261-1000
Ferre by Ferre	Ferre/Gary Farn, Ltd.	(203) 878-8900
Fiamma	Halston Borghese	(212) 572-3100
Fidji	Guy Laroche	(800) 422-2360
First	Van Cleef & Arpels/Sanofi	(212) 230-0500
Fleur de Fleurs	Nina Ricci Parfums	(212) 230-0500
Fleurs d'Elle	Classic Fragrances Ltd.	(212) 929-2266
Fleurs de Rocaille	Caron/Jean Patou	(212) 688-5568
Folavril	Annick Goutal	(212) 759-0650
4711	Muelhens	(203) 787-4711
Fracas	Piguet/Alfin	(212) 333-7700
Fred Hayman's Touch	Fred Hayman Beverly Hills	(310) 271-3100
Gabriela Sabatini	Muelhens	(203) 787-4711
Galanos	Galanos/Gary Farn Ltd.	(203) 878-8900
Galore	Monteil/Lancaster Group	(212) 593-7400
Gardenia	Chanel	(212) 688-5055
Gardénia Passion	Annick Goutal	(212) 759-0650
Gem	Van Cleef & Arpels/Sanofi	(212) 230-0500
Genny Shine	Gary Farn, Ltd.	(203) 878-8900
Gianfranco Ferre	Ferre/Gary Farn, Ltd.	(203) 878-8900
Giorgio Beverly Hills	Giorgio Beverly Hills/Avon	(310) 453-0711
Giò	Armani/Cosmair	(212) 818-1500
Givenchy III	Parfums Givenchy	(212) 759-7566
Golconda	Classic Fragrances Ltd.	(212) 929-2266
Gucci No. 1	Gucci/Muelhens	(203) 787-4711
Gucci No. 3	Gucci/Muelhens	(203) 787-4711
Guess?	Guess?/Revlon	(212) 527-4000
Habanita	Molinard/Classic Fragrances	(212) 929-2266
Halston	Halston Borghese	(212) 572-3100
Heure Exquise	Annick Goutal	(212) 759-0650

Histoire d'Amour	French Fragrances	(305) 624-7849
Hot	Blass/Revlon	(212) 527-4000
Ice Water by Pino Silvestre	Classic Fragrances Ltd.	(212) 929-2266
Il Bacio	Halston Borghese	(212) 572-3100
Infini	Caron/Jean Patou	(212) 688-5568
Isis	Wm. Owen Fragrances	(407) 833-4076
Ivoire	Balmain/Alfin	(212) 333-7700
Jardins de Bagatelle	Guerlain	(212) 751-1870
Je Reviens	Model Imperial Fine Fragrances	(407) 241-8244
Jean-Paul Gaultier	No N. American distributor at print time	
Jessica McClintock	Jessica McClintock	(415) 495-3030
Jicky	Guerlain	(212) 751-1870
Jil Sander No. 4	Lancaster Group	(212) 593-7400
Jolie Madame	Balmain/Alfin	(212) 333-7700
Joop! pour Femmes	Lancaster Group	(212) 593-7400
Joy	Jean Patou	(212) 688-5568
K de Krizia	Krizia/Gary Farn, Ltd.	(203) 878-8900
KL	Parfums International	(212) 261-1000
Knowing	Estée Lauder	(212) 572-4200
L'Air du Temps	Nina Ricci Parfums	(212) 230-0500
L'Arte de Gucci	Gucci/Muelhens	(203) 787-4711
L'Heure Attendue (Ma Collect'n)	Jean Patou	(212) 688-5568
L'Heure Bleue	Guerlain	(212) 751-1870
L'Insolent	Jourdan/Muelhens	(203) 787-4711
L'Interdit	Parfums Givenchy	(212) 759-7566
La Prairie	La Prairie	(212) 459-1600
Laguna	Dali/Fine Fragrances	(305) 624-7849
Lalique	Sanofi Beaute	(212) 230-0500
Laura Ashley No. 1	Ashley/Alfin	(212) 333-7700
Lauren	Ralph Lauren/Cosmair	(212) 818-1500
Le Dix	Balenciaga/Fragrance Group	(212) 557-8177
Les Fleurs de Claude Monet	Muelhens	(203) 787-4711
Léonard de Léonard	Léonard/Jean Pax	(305) 593-0982
Listen	H. Alpert & Co.	(310) 478-0222
Liu	Guerlain	(212) 751-1870
Liz Claiborne	Liz Claiborne Cosmetics	(212) 354-4900
Lumière	Rochas/Jean Patou	(212) 688-5568
Lutéce	Parquet/Houbigant	(201) 941-3400
Ma Collection	Jean Patou	(212) 688-5568
Ma Griffe	Model Imperial Fine Fragrances	(407) 241-8244
Ma Liberté	Jean Patou	(212) 688-5568
Mackie, Bob Mackie	Mackie/Riviera Concepts	(213) 658-7864
Mad Moments	Madeleine Mono	(516) 287-3385
Madame Rochas	Jean Patou	(212) 688-5568
Madeleine de Madeleine	Madeleine Mono	(516) 287-3385
Mademoiselle Ricci	Nina Ricci Parfums	(212) 230-0500
Magic Noire	Lancôme/Cosmair	(212) 818-1500
Magnetic	Muelhens	(203) 787-4711
Maroussia	No N. American distributor at print time	
Maud Frizon Parfum	Maud Frizon	(212) 249-5368
Michelle	Balenciaga/Fragrance Group	(212) 557-8177
Miss Balmain	Balmain/Alfin	(212) 333-7700
Miss Dior	Christian Dior Perfumes	(212) 418-0400
Mitsouko	Guerlain	(212) 751-1870
Molinard de Molinard	Molinard/Classic Fragrances	(212) 929-2266
Moment Suprême (Ma Collection)	Jean Patou	(212) 688-5568

Moments Priscilla Presley	Presley/Muelhens	(203) 787-4711
Moods	Krizia/Gary Farn, Ltd.	(203) 878-8900
Moschino	Moschino/H. Alpert & Co.	(310) 478-0222
Must de Cartier	Parfums Cartier	(212) 753-0111
Mystère	Rochas/Jean Patou	(212) 688-5568
Nahema	Guerlain	(212) 751-1870
Narcisse Noir	Caron/Jean Patou	(212) 688-5568
Nicole Miller	Miller/Riviera Concepts	(213) 658-7864
Niki de Saint Phalle	Alfin	(212) 333-7700
Nina	Nina Ricci Parfums	(212) 230-0500
Niro 15	Niro	(214) 321-9352
Niro 119	Niro	(214) 321-9352
Nocturnes	Caron/Jean Patou	(212) 688-5568
Noir for Women by P. Morabito	Classic Fragrances Ltd.	(212) 929-2266
Norell	Revlon	(212) 527-4000
Normandie (Ma Collection)	Jean Patou	(212) 688-5568
Nude	Blass/Revlon	(212) 527-4000
Nuit de Noël	Caron/Jean Patou	(212) 688-5568
Obsession	Calvin Klein Cosmetics	(212) 759-8888
Odalisque	Classic Fragrances Ltd.	(212) 929-2266
Oh la la!	MacFarlane & Associates	(914) 639-9170
Ombre Rose	Jean Philippe	(212) 983-2640
One Perfect Rose	Georgette Mosbacher	(212) 288-7345
1000 de Jean Patou	Jean Patou	(212) 688-5568
One Unlimited Perfume	La Parfumerie Inc.	(212) 750-1111
Opium	Yves Saint Laurent	(212) 621-7300
Oscar de la Renta	De la Renta/Sanofi Beaute	(212) 230-0500
Paloma Picasso	Picasso/Cosmair	(212) 818-1500
Panthère	Parfums Cartier	(212) 753-0111
Parfum d'Hermès	Hermes Parfums	(212) 759-7585
Parfum Sacré	Caron/Jean Patou	(212) 688-5568
Paris	Yves Saint Laurent	(212) 621-7300
Parure	Guerlain	(212) 751-1870
Passion	Annick Goutal	(212) 759-0650
Pavlova	Muelhens	(203) 787-4711
Pheromone	Marilyn Miglin	(312) 943-1120
Poison	Christian Dior Perfumes	(212) 418-0400
Prélude	Balenciaga/Fragrance Group	(212) 557-8177
Private Collection	Estée Lauder	(212) 572-4200
Quadrille	Balenciaga/Fragrance Group	(212) 557-8177
Quartz	French Fragrances	(305) 624-7849
Que sais-je? (Ma Collection)	Jean Patou	(212) 688-5568
Quelques Fleurs L'Original	Parfums Houbigant Paris	(201) 945-2666
Raffinée	Parfums Houbigant Paris	(201) 945-2666
Realities	Liz Claiborne Cosmetics	(212) 354-4900
Realm	Erox Corporation	(212) 758-9797
Red Door	Elizabeth Arden Co.	(212) 261-1350
Red	Giorgio Beverly Hills	(310) 453-0711
Reverie	Wm. Owen Fragrances	(407) 833-4076
Rive Gauche	Yves Saint Laurent	(212) 621-7300
Roma	Biagiotti/Eurocos U.S.A.	(800) 572-3232
Romeo Gigli	Gigli/H. Alpert & Co.	(310) 478-0222
Rose Absolue	Annick Goutal	(212) 759-0650
Rose Cardin	Cardin/Tsumura International	(201) 223-9000
Royal Secret	Monteil/Lancaster Group	(212) 593-7400
Rumba	Balenciaga/Fragrance Group	(212) 557-8177

Safari	Ralph Lauren/Cosmair	(212) 818-1500
Salvador Dali	Dali/Fine Fragrances	(305) 624-7849
Samsara	Guerlain	(212) 751-1870
Scaasi	Tsumura International	(210) 319-3900
Scherrer 2	Elizabeth Arden	(212) 261-1000
Secret of Venus	Classic Fragrances Ltd.	(212) 929-2266
Senso	Ungaro Parfums	(212) 303-5920
Shalimar	Guerlain	(212) 751-1870
Smalto Donna	Parlux Fragrances	(305) 946-7700
Society by Burberrys	Alfin	(212) 333-7700
Spellbound	Estée Lauder	(212) 572-4200
Spoiled	Theodore of Beverly Hills	(310) 278-4130
Sublime	Jean Patou	(212) 688-5568
Sunflowers	Elizabeth Arden Co.	(212) 261-1350
Sung, Alfred Sung	Sung/Riviera Concepts	(213) 658-7864
Sweet Courrèges	Courrèges/Jean Pax	(305) 593-0982
Tamango	Léonard//Jean Pax	(305) 593-0982
Tatiana	Diane Von Furstenberg	(212) 753-1111
Teatro alla Scala	Krizia/Gary Farn, Ltd.	(203) 878-8900
Tendre Poison	Christian Dior Perfumes	(212) 418-0400
Tianne	Classic Fragrances Ltd.	(212) 929-2266
Tiffany	Tiffany	(212) 755-8000
Trésor	Lancôme/Cosmair	(212) 818-1500
Tribù	Benetton Cosmetics Corp.	(212) 832-6616
Tubéreuse	Annick Goutal	(212) 759-0650
Tuscany Per Donna	Aramis/Estée Lauder	(212) 572-4200
273 for Women	Fred Hayman Beverly Hills	(310) 271-3100
Un Jour	Jourdan/Muelhens	(203) 787-4711
Ungaro	Ungaro Parfums	(212) 303-5920
V'E Versace	Versace/Vepro U.S.A.	(212) 935-4800
Vacances (Ma Collection)	Jean Patou	(212) 688-5568
Van Cleef & Arpels	Van Cleef & Arpels/Sanofi	(212) 230-0500
Vanderbilt	Vanderbilt/Cosmair	(212) 818-1500
Vendetta	Valentino/Parfums International	(212) 261-1000
Venezia	Biagiotti/Eurocos U.S.A.	(800) 572-3232
Vent Vert	Balmain/Alfin	(212) 333-7700
Versus for Women	Versace/Vepro U.S.A.	(212) 935-4800
Vicky Tiel	Parlux Fragrances	(305) 946-7700
Vivid	Liz Claiborne Cosmetics	(212) 354-4900
Vol de Nuit	Guerlain	(212) 751-1870
Volcan D'Amour	Diane Von Furstenberg	(212) 753-1111
Volupté	De la Renta/Sanofi Beaute	(212) 230-0500
Vôtre	Jourdan/Muelhens	(203) 787-4711
Weil de Weil	Weil/Classic Fragrances	(212) 929-2266
White Diamonds	Taylor/Parfums International	(212) 261-1000
White Linen	Estée Lauder	(212) 572-4200
White Shoulders	Parfums International	(212) 261-1000
Wings	Giorgio Beverly Hills	(310) 453-0711
...with Love	Fred Hayman Beverly Hills	(310) 271-3100
Womenswear by A. Julian	Paul Sebastian	(908) 493-4499
Wrappings	Clinique Laboratories	(212) 572-3800
Y	Yves Saint Laurent	(212) 621-7300
Youth Dew	Estée Lauder	(212) 572-4200
Ysatis	Parfums Givenchy	(212) 759-7566
Zarolia	Barclay Perfumes	(908) 459-4921
Zibeline	Classic Fragrances Ltd.	(212) 929-2266

To order more copies of *Fabulous Fragrances* or to be placed on our mailing list, send postcard, call or fax.

Name

Company

Address

City/State/Zip/Country

Phone (If we have questions about your order)

Please send _____ (mark quantity) copies of *Fabulous Fragrances* at $29 ($U.S.) each $ _____

Please send _____ (mark quantity) copies of *Fabulous Fragrances For Men* at $29 ($U.S.) each $ _____

Please send _____ (mark quantity) sets of Fabulous Fragrances™ Perfume Wardrobe Sampler at $25 ($U.S.) each $ _____

California residents add 8.25 % sales tax $ _____

Please add $5.50 shipping and handling for each item $ _____

Please add $8.50 shipping and handling for each item outside of U.S. $ _____

TOTAL $ _____

☐ Check or money order enclosed. Make check payable to: Crescent House Publishing.

CRESCENT HOUSE PUBLISHING, P.O. BOX 16724, BEVERLY HILLS, CA 90209, TEL: (310) 364-0551 • FAX: (310) 274-0717

☐ Visa/Mastercard Account# ☐☐☐☐☐☐☐☐☐☐☐☐☐☐☐☐

Expiration Date: _____ Signature _____

☐ I'm not ordering now, but please put me on your mailing list.

For orders of 10 or more copies of Fabulous Fragrances, inquire about our corporate rates. Call (310) 364-0551.

To order more copies of *Fabulous Fragrances* or to be placed on our mailing list, send postcard, call or fax.

Name

Company

Address

City/State/Zip/Country

Phone (If we have questions about your order)

Please send _____ (mark quantity) copies of *Fabulous Fragrances* at $29 ($U.S.) each $ _____

Please send _____ (mark quantity) copies of *Fabulous Fragrances For Men* at $29 ($U.S.) each $ _____

Please send _____ (mark quantity) sets of Fabulous Fragrances™ Perfume Wardrobe Sampler at $25 ($U.S.) each $ _____

California residents add 8.25 % sales tax $ _____

Please add $5.50 shipping and handling for each item $ _____

Please add $8.50 shipping and handling for each item outside of U.S. $ _____

TOTAL $ _____

☐ Check or money order enclosed. Make check payable to: Crescent House Publishing.

CRESCENT HOUSE PUBLISHING, P.O. BOX 16724, BEVERLY HILLS, CA 90209, TEL: (310) 364-0551 • FAX: (310) 274-0717

☐ Visa/Mastercard Account# ☐☐☐☐☐☐☐☐☐☐☐☐☐☐☐☐

Expiration Date: _____ Signature _____

☐ I'm not ordering now, but please put me on your mailing list.

For orders of 10 or more copies of Fabulous Fragrances, inquire about our corporate rates. Call (310) 364-0551.